MW01126107

Praise for *Seasonal Living with Herbs*

"Jess beautifully welcomes us into her botanical sanctuary, sharing her personal journey into gardening and herbalism, a realm filled with insights cultivated through hands-on experience. *Seasonal Living with Herbs* is not only a practical guide to gardening, but an invitation to add intention to your life by embracing the rhythms of nature. Readers will be drawn into the visually alluring pages and stick around for the how-to growing and harvesting tips, informative plant guides, and the thoughtful collection of herbal recipes and projects."

—Amber Meyers, co-director of the Herbal Academy

"In this book, Jess weaves together words and herbs in inspiring ways, igniting the reader's love and curiosity for the wonderful world of green and growing things. Peppered with creative projects and stunning photography, flipping through these pages feels like sitting down for tea in Jess's garden, surrounded by beautiful blooms and the buzzing of pollinators."

—Catarina Seixas, author of *The Wild Craft*

"Jess does a lovely job of capturing the many beneficial aspects of gardening not only for oneself, but the environment in which the garden grows. She touches eloquently on subjects of tending to one's mental health, making a sanctuary for beloved pollinators, and all aspects in between. This book paints a beautiful year-round portrait of just how delightful gardening can be."

—Lauren May, Must Love Herbs

"Through her lens and her experiential knowledge, Jess shares creative and beautiful ways to weave plants into your everyday garden, kitchen, and home."

—Alyson Morgan, folk herbalist and author of *Our Kindred Home*

"This book is an invitation to observe and tap into the nurturing and healing power of plants, shared in down-to-earth, accessible language that will empower you to deepen your relationship with the natural world. Whether your passion for plants is just sprouting or you're already deep into your herbalism journey, this is a must have for any nature lover's shelf."

—Dagny Kream, The Cottage Peach

Seasonal Living *with* Herbs

Seasonal Living *with* Herbs

How to Grow, Harvest, Preserve and Use Herbs Year Round

Jess Buttermore

yellow pear press

CORAL GABLES

For permission requests, please contact the publisher at:
Mango Publishing Group
2850 S Douglas Road, 2nd Floor
Coral Gables, FL 33134 USA
info@mango.bz

For special orders, quantity sales, course adoptions and corporate sales, please email the publisher at sales@mango.bz. For trade and wholesale sales, please contact Ingram Publisher Services at customer.service@ingramcontent.com or +1.800.509.4887.

Seasonal Living with Herbs: How to Grow, Harvest, Preserve and Use Herbs Year Round

Library of Congress Cataloging-in-Publication number: 2023945345
ISBNs: (hc) 978-1-68481-353-7 (pb) 978-1-68481-354-4 (e) 978-1-68481-355-1
BISAC category code: GAR009000, GARDENING / Herbs

Printed in the United States of America

Table of Contents

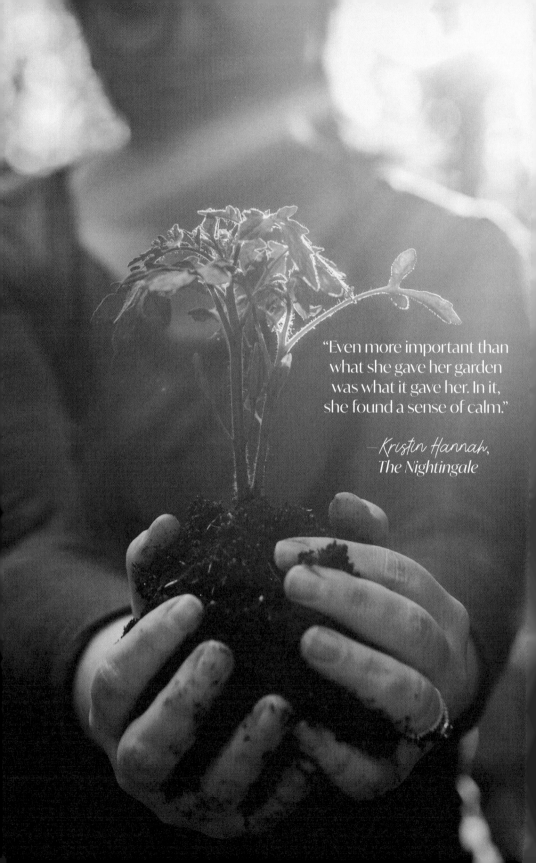

"Even more important than what she gave her garden was what it gave her. In it, she found a sense of calm."

—Kristin Hannah,
The Nightingale

Introduction

An Herbal Awakening

For me, the gardening cycle begins in the greenhouse. With each seed sown, new ideas are budding. New dreams for what the coming year's garden will hold and how I might inspire others to grow alongside me. Beginning in January, I can be found in my greenhouse growing hundreds of herbs and flowers from seed, nurturing tiny seedlings into robust plants that can be planted out as soon as that final frost has passed. And for the six months following that, my garden is blooming with flowers and herbs. The more time I spend in it, the more I realize how important gardens have become to us over the past few years. Gardens are no longer simply a place to grow plants. They have taken on a more holistic purpose for many of us, playing a vital role in both our physical health and mental wellbeing. It was this realization that led me to begin documenting my gardening journey.

9

I learned very quickly that fellow gardeners and herbalists are extremely generous with their knowledge and insight, and it didn't take long for me to realize that I wanted to pay that same courtesy forward by sharing my knowledge and experiences of gardening through my words, my land, and my lens. I turned my focus, and ultimately my business, toward sharing my journey in gardening, herbalism, and botanical design with others by writing about and photographing what I was learning. When the opportunity was presented to me to compile all my experiences, insight, recipes, tutorials, and photography into a book, I was ecstatic. As a professional photographer, photographing herbs and flowers that I've grown from seed is one of the ways I show gratitude for them and the memories they make for my family. Gratitude for the lands and the means to grown them. And for the beautiful space in which to enjoy them. Photography is my way of preserving them long beyond their vase or jar life. I came to realize that this book was something I had been working toward for years without recognizing it. Each garden design, seed choice, photograph, and blog article were steppingstones toward the book you hold in your hands.

Is there any better way to feel connected to the earth then to grow and tend to a garden filled with herbs? You give it time, patience, energy, and attention, and in return, it gives you buckets full of medicinal and culinary herbs and a place to turn your thoughts. My garden breathes new purpose nearly every time I visit it. Being outdoors in my garden, surrounded by the botanicals I've nurtured from seed, not only balances my brain chemistry, but it also has a beautiful way of pulling me away from the confines and stresses of modern technology. It is my dwelling place for creativity. My sanctuary and refuge. The flowers and herbs I cultivate in my garden have a secret language all their own. It's just a matter of slowing down long enough to hear it.

As a garden grows, so does the gardener grow alongside it because the garden is very much a teacher. It has taught me patience, persistence, and mindfulness. A series of traumatic events unfolded in my life as a young adult, leading to the onset of panic attacks and severe anxiety. Gardening has helped lessen the symptoms associated with my anxiety and the burdens that weigh heavy on my heart. There are always more pressing things to do, but time in the garden provides the sustenance I need to do those other things well. Even today, as my garden feels less like a new adventure and more like an old friend, it continues to shape, steady, and inspire me. It whispers to my heart and encourages me to stop and enjoy the present. I no longer wish for the next mile of my journey but rather enjoy the path I'm on at this very moment. I truly believe I am a better wife, mother, daughter, friend and neighbor thanks to this space and the joy it has brought me.

One of the things I love most about herbs, is that no matter how my garden evolves over the years, there's always a place for them. Herbs have transformed my botanical story, flawlessly intermingling with my flowers as the perfect little companions in the most enchanting way. I take great pride in designing my garden each year, tending to it, and preserving its bountiful harvests. I find even the simplest tasks, like snipping a few quick sprigs of this or that herb when I'm preparing a meal or craft cocktail, equally as gratifying. My hope is that the pages that follow will become a resource to you, inspiring you to grow a garden filled with herbs, and guiding you through that process. This book explores my personal experiences growing a holistic herb and flower garden and, alongside it, growing in my relationship with the earth. May the insight, guidance, and imagery filling these pages inspire you to begin (or continue on) your journey with herbs. To understand them. To grow them. To fall in love with them. And to incorporate them into your garden and daily life in meaningful ways. Consider this book your personal invitation to grow with me.

Within These Pages

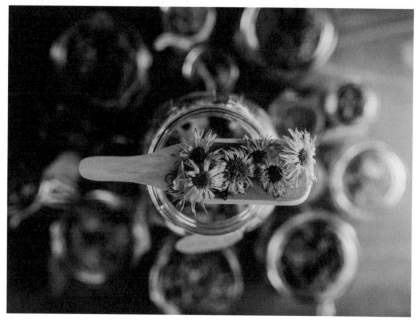

"If you look the right way,
you can see that the whole world is a garden."

—Frances Hodgson Burnett,
The Secret Garden (1849–1924)

Part I of this book introduces herb gardening from an approachable perspective, walking you through important considerations when establishing an herb garden, from choosing what to grow and considering the environmental impacts of these choices, to sowing seeds and nurturing seedlings.

Part II takes you through my processes for harvesting herbs and propagating cuttings, and various ways to preserve herbs for culinary, medicinal and crafting purposes. I also share my checklist for winterizing my herb garden.

In Part III, I dig deeper into some of the herbs I grow in my backyard garden with diverse beneficial uses. As we become familiar with their properties and uses, we add a layer of depth to our understanding of their powers. This section also walks you through how to care for, harvest, and preserve each highlighted herb.

Nature is cyclical. In fact, its predictability is one of the very things I love most about it. Nature speaks to us through all the botanical gifts of each season. We look forward to them. We prepare for them. We appreciate the seasons for all that they are, time and time again. They give us hope and consistency, yet cannot be rushed. Each season delivers in its own perfect time. The fourth section of the book takes you on an herbal journey following the earthly, botanically driven calendar. It is filled with recipes, techniques, tutorials, and projects that feed my soul during each season of the year, sharing how I use herbs in my home in practical and interesting ways that exercise creativity.

Woven through the book are botanically themed and literary quotes, many which are from the Victorian era. Victorians had a deep appreciation for the beauty and usefulness of herbs, and I wanted to honor that as part of my herbal storytelling. An herbal glossary is also included at the back of the book so that you can conveniently source content about a specific herb. May these pages welcome you into the seasonal cycle of nature and remind you to never underestimate the healing, stabilizing, restorative power of a garden filled with herbs.

Important Note: While medicinal herbs can be helpful in many ways, they should always be used with caution and under the guidance of your healthcare professional. The author and publisher of this book makes no medical claims to diagnose or treat medical conditions. Readers must do their own research concerning the safety and usage of herbs.

Reconnecting with Our Roots

"A shared appreciation of a subject or a mutual way of life is the best way to seal a friendship."

—*Rosemary Verey*, *A Countrywoman's Year* (1918–2001)

A Brief History of Herb Gardening

The history of herb gardening is rich and fascinating, filled with the wisdom and traditions of cultures long past. Archeological studies have suggested that the practice of herbalism for medicinal purposes dates as far back as 60,000 years ago in Iraq and 8,000 years ago in China. Records dating back 5,000 years to the Sumerians have described humans cultivating herbs for culinary, medicinal, and spiritual purposes, and the practice has remained an important part of our lives ever since.

Herbalism was well-documented by the ancient Egyptians beginning in 3000 BC, who cultivated herb gardens, had schools dedicated to herbalism, and used herbs in their embalming rituals. They used herbs to flavor their food, to make cosmetics and perfumes, and to treat pain and skin irritations. Thyme, aloe, cannabis, fennel, and juniper were among the most widely used herbs of that time.

The Greeks and Romans used herbs for culinary, medicinal, and religious purposes as well. During the Middle Ages, monasteries became centers for herb gardening, and herbal remedies were developed to treat a wide range of ailments. As part of running the household, medieval women were often responsible for growing and harvesting herbs for a variety of purposes. The herbs were also preserved to provide vitamins and nutrients to their family members during the winter months when fresh herbs were not available. Before modern medicine, these herbs were often the difference between life and death. Some of the most commonly used herbs during the Middle Ages were lavender, rosemary, sage, and peppermint.

Hundreds of tribal cultures have been using both wild and cultivated herbs for medicinal and culinary purposes for thousands of years, which continue to be a vital part of their culture and way of life today. Each tribe has its own traditions and herbal knowledge, which is passed down from generation to generation. Native American tribes used herbs to treat illnesses, underlying health conditions, and injuries. They also used herbs for culinary and spiritual purposes. Some of the most common herbs used by Native Americans are cedar, sage, echinacea, mint, yarrow, and sweetgrass.

During the Renaissance, herb gardening became more of an art form, with gardens designed to be aesthetically pleasing as well as functional. Famous artists and intellectuals, such as Leonardo da Vinci and Michelangelo, grew herbs in their gardens, and the use of herbs in cooking continued to be an important part of daily life. In fact, formal garden designs today are often developed to preserve the garden heritage of this era, filled with the herbs that were most widely used during the reign of Queen Victoria. It was also during this time that herbs and flowers were used to symbolize emotions and messages, thus forming what is now known as the language of flowers. Some of the most popular herbs from the Victorian era were bee balm, catmint, chamomile, dill, lavender, lemon balm, rose, and rosemary. This truly was an intriguing period with a rich botanical history. If you would like to learn more about Victorian botanical symbolism, as well as how to infuse bouquets with meaning, I encourage you to explore my book, *The Love Language of Flowers*.

If I could go back in time and walk one garden, it would be Claude Monet's in Giverny, France. Though Monet is most widely known as a brilliant impressionistic artist, he considered his garden his most beautiful

15

work. He was a skilled horticulturalist who was constantly incorporating new plants into his garden to add texture and color, in much the same way he added paint to canvas. Although it was carefully planned, it had a wild natural look to it that I admire and try to emulate in my own garden design and he, too, loved intermingling herbs with colorful flowers.

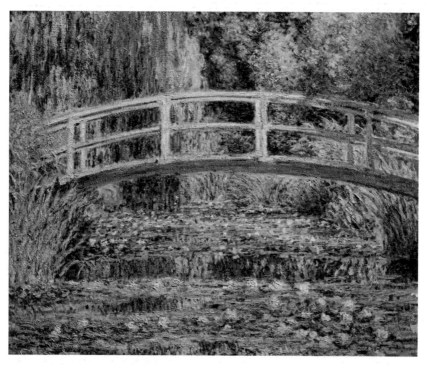

Bridge over a Pond of Water Lilies oil on canvas, 1899, by Claude Monet

As time went on, herb gardening became more widely practiced, with more and more people around the world recognizing the value of herbs in their lives. Many herbs are perennials, and herbs can often be divided and tend to be rather low-maintenance, needing no more than regular watering, occasional fertilizing, and annual trimming. Today, herb gardening is a beloved tradition that continues to be taught and passed down through generations. It's a way to connect with the earth and with the wisdom of our ancestors and stands as a reminder of the continuously healing power of nature.

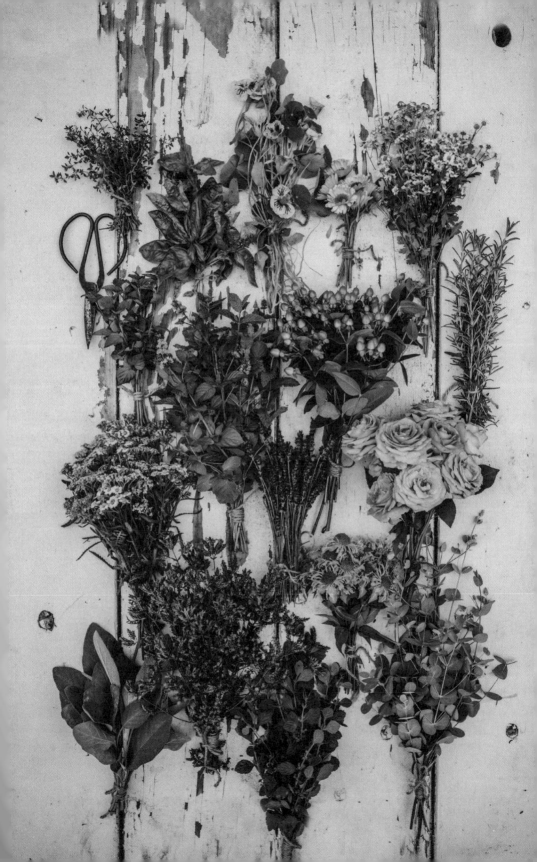

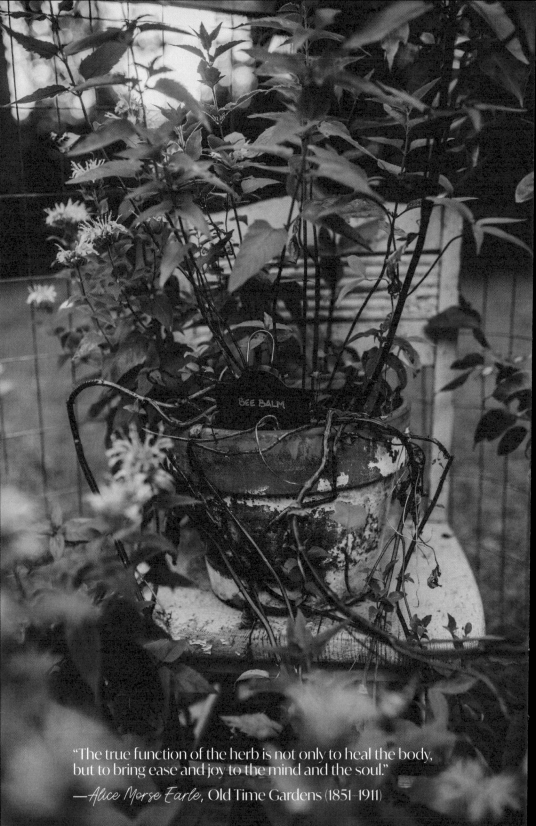

"The true function of the herb is not only to heal the body, but to bring ease and joy to the mind and the soul."

—*Alice Morse Earle*, Old Time Gardens (1851–1911)

A Garden for the Mind, Body, and Soul

"The glory of gardening: hands in the dirt,
head in the sun, heart with nature. To nurture a
garden is to feed not just the body, but the soul."

—*Alfred Austin*, English poet (1835–1913)

In much the same way that holistic medicine takes into account mental and social factors in addition to symptoms of an illness to treat the whole person, holistic gardening is an approach that benefits the mind, spirit, and body of the gardener. Gardening has many benefits that can improve your overall health and well-being. It's truly remarkable how working in the garden, with your hands in the soil, can alter the balance of neurotransmitters in your brain, relieving stress and anxiousness. If I hadn't experienced it firsthand, I'm not sure I'd believe it. In a garden of herbs, one can find a sanctuary of peace and a place of solace where worries ease. Let's dig into the multitude of benefits of gardening.

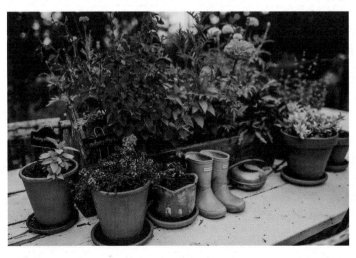

Physical Benefits of Gardening

"It was such a pleasure to sink one's hands into the warm earth, to feel at one's fingertips the possibilities of the new season."

— *Kate Morton*, The Forgotten Garden

Let's start with the obvious. From digging to planting, weeding to watering, gardening requires a significant amount of physical movement that can help you stay active, burn calories, and improve flexibility and strength. It can also improve cardiovascular health by lowering blood pressure and reducing the risk of heart disease. Gardening has also been associated with a reduced risk of chronic diseases such as obesity, diabetes, and cancer.

Spending time in nature and engaging in physical activity through gardening can help improve sleep quality and reduce the risk of sleep disorders. It has also been shown to reduce stress levels and promote relaxation, which can have a positive impact on your physical health. Some medicinal herbs can also help boost the immune system, which can help prevent illness.

Being exposed to dirt and soil in your garden can help boost your immune system and increase your resistance to certain diseases. It's true! The smell of wet earth, known as geosmin, is released through the activity of soil bacteria called actinomycetes, and has a pleasing and soothing effect on most people.

By growing herbs in your garden, you are surrounding yourself with botanicals that ignite all the senses: beautiful blooms as far as the eye can see, the sweet fragrances of herbs in the breeze, interesting textures to feel as you're harvesting, varieties of flavors to taste along the way, and slowing down to listen to the song of the pollinators around you.

Mental Benefits of Gardening

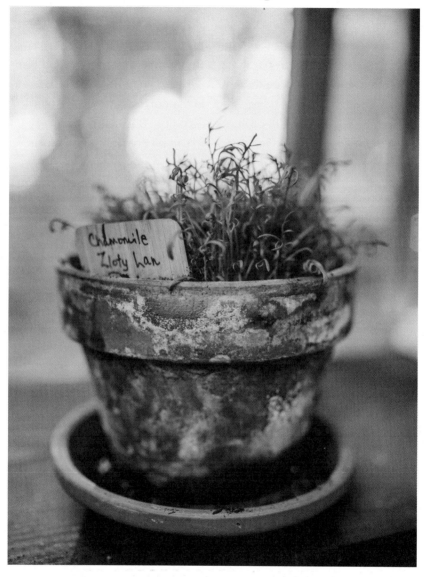

"A garden is always the expression of someone's mind and the outcome of someone's care."

—*Sue Stuart-Smith*, *The Well-Gardened Mind*

Gardening has been shown to improve mood by increasing levels of neurotransmitters like endorphins and dopamine, as well as serotonin. It can also help reduce symptoms of depression and anxiety, and provide a sense of purpose and fulfillment, positively impacting overall mental health. Herbal preparations from your garden add another layer of depth to the mental health benefits, as certain medicinal herbs have been found to have a calming effect on the nervous system, helping reduce anxiety and further promote relaxation. Because gardening requires focus and attention to detail, it can be considered helpful in promoting mindfulness and reducing negative thoughts.

There is a deep sense of accomplishment that comes with gardening. Gardeners take great pride in their dedicated growing space, as well as in harvesting the plants they worked so hard to germinate, nurture, and grow. Harvesting herbs and blooms and using them in your home and kitchen is a very rewarding and empowering experience.

The garden can be a reprieve from the busyness of life, and being surrounded by nature has been found to have a range of mental health benefits. Spending time in a garden space has also been proven helpful to people recovering from post-traumatic stress disorder (PTSD). In *The Well-Gardened Mind*, Stuart-Smith shares that garden spaces naturally bring the body to a lower level of physiological arousal by slowing the heart rate within minutes of entering them. It is also believed that the color green strikes the eye in such a way that it requires no adjustment, therefore lowering a person's level of arousal. Within twenty to thirty minutes, those in garden spaces have reduced levels of the stress hormone cortisol.

Documenting the details of your herb garden through garden journaling is another calming, therapeutic activity that can improve mental health. Journaling about your gardening experiences can help you prioritize challenges you experience along the way and provides a place to document the solutions so that you know how to combat them next time. It can also help you track daily tasks and boost your confidence by listing successes you experience along the way. Garden journaling can also include drawing, another soothing, calming activity that lowers your heart rate and stabilizes your breathing pattern. My personal garden journal includes sketches, notes organized by month, and a list of plants I will and won't grow next year. I often bring my journal down to the garden with me so I can record my thoughts as I care for and harvest in each bed.

Emotional Benefits of Gardening

"To garden is to nurture
and to be nurtured simultaneously."

—The Herbal Academy

Gardens provide a gathering place with a welcoming atmosphere where you can spend time with those you care about. Growing flowers and herbs and harvesting them to be appreciated indoors helps make your home a beautiful, soothing environment that promotes happiness. Furthermore, giving the gift of herbs is good for the soul, bringing joy and health benefits both to the botanical gift giver as well as the recipient.

A Tapestry of Color

A significant amount of research exists exploring the relationship between color and mood. The findings suggest that color can impact physiological responses such as heart rate, blood pressure and body temperature, as well as emotional responses such as excitement or calmness. Just as different colors elicit different emotions and moods, so do plants of those colors. Here is a list of my favorite herbs organized into color categories along with the mood that color stimulates so that you may consider adding your favorite colors and emotions into your garden:

Red is often associated with passion, energy, and excitement. (But be careful, as it is also associated with warning, eliciting a feeling of panic, anger, or danger.) To incorporate splashes of red in your herb garden, consider growing red varieties of bee balm, rose, poppy, and scarlet (crimson) sage.

Pink is often associated with love, romance, and femininity. Add pink to your herb garden with pink varieties of creeping thyme, bee balm, rose, and yarrow. Soapwort and motherwort have pink blossoms, as do certain varieties of hibiscus, hyssop, echinacea, and sweet marjoram. I'm also completely smitten with ornamental oregano and its lime to pink ombre cascading bracts that are everlasting when dried.

Orange is a warm and welcoming color that can create a sense of enthusiasm and excitement. It is often used in advertisements to promote a fun and energetic vibe. Marigold is possibly the most commonly recognized orange-flowering herb, with calendula, nasturtium, and California and Iceland poppy following close behind. There are also gorgeous varieties of rose and echinacea in beautiful cantaloupe and vibrant orange hues that are worth noting.

24

Yellow is most often associated with happiness, optimism, and positivity. To incorporate yellow in your herb garden, consider growing chamomile, dandelion, dill, fennel, goldenrod, tarragon, tansy and St. John's wort, however I prefer to include rarer yellow-flowering herbs in softer hues like Ivory Princess calendula and Moonlight marigold. There are also beautiful buttery yellow varieties of rose, nasturtium and echinacea that are sure to catch your eye.

White, often associated with cleanliness, purity, safety, and innocence, is one of the most common herb blooming colors. Most notable are chamomile, feverfew, yarrow, rose, and garlic chive. Coriander and chickweed also flower white, and the pillows of meadowsweet are always eye-catching. Less common options include elder, sweet woodruff, caraway, and anise.

Green is fittingly associated with nature, growth, and balance and nearly every herb has green foliage. My favorite shades of green are the creamy greens of eucalyptus and the soft powdery greens of common garden sage.

Blue is often associated with calmness, serenity, and trust. I couldn't imagine my garden without my favorite blue herb, borage. Rosemary, hyssop, chicory, and butterfly pea flower are other lovely blue additions to any garden. Lastly, I obsess over Blue Shrimp honeywort and hope to grow it someday.

Purple, most often associated with creativity, luxury, and royalty, is another staple color in my garden, next to pink. My favorite purple herbs include lavender, blossoms of chive, purple basil, giant lavender hyssop, clary sage, lilac, sweet marjoram, honeywort, and bee balm. My list of purple herbs would not be complete without including traditional echinacea, giant lavender hyssop, rose, and the blossoms of sage, lemon balm, thyme, rosemary, spearmint, and oregano.

In the same way that each gardener has a different preference for herbal flavors and fragrances, the colors of the herbs you incorporate into your garden space is also an individual preference. Consider your favorite colors as well as colors that are influenced by personal experiences in your life or cultural background. Keep in mind, also, flowers you may be growing alongside your herbs and what colors of herbs would best coordinate with those blooms for ornamental purposes and floral design.

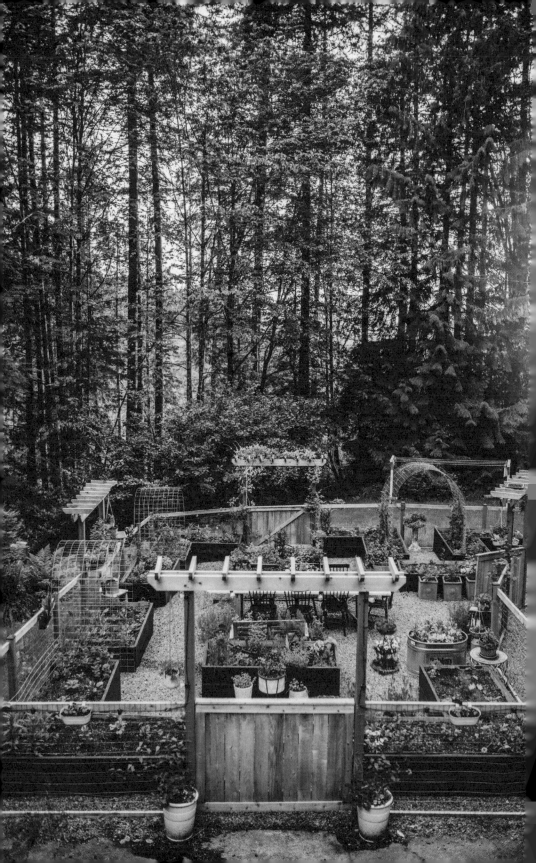

Part I
Grow + Tend

"To plant a garden is to believe in tomorrow."
—Audrey Hepburn (1929–1993)

Building the Foundation

Here are some considerations when establishing an herb garden.

Sunlight

Herbs need sufficient sunlight, so choose a location to build your herb garden (or place containers) that gets at least six to eight hours of direct sunlight every day. For example, some of the most common herbs that thrive in full sun include basil, calendula, chamomile, dill, fennel, lavender, nasturtium, rosemary, and summer savory. Part-sun herbs, such as basil, lemon balm, cilantro, chive, mint, and parsley will thrive in three to six hours of sunlight daily and prefer to be protected from harsh mid-day sun during hot summer days. To measure the amount of sun in a particular space, observe sunlight exposure beginning just after sunrise through to sunset. Take note of areas of the space that never get full sun (are shaded due to trees or structures) or that have filtered or dappled sunlight due to tree shadows. The longer and brighter the sun shines in the space you are considering, the more flexibility you will have in which herbs you will have success growing. Generally speaking, south-facing gardens, porches, balconies and windowsills get the most sun exposure.

Purpose

Consider the purpose of your herb garden. Will it be a quiet place you go to find solitude away from the hustle and bustle of everyday life? Or will it be strictly for practical purposes? If the former, consider arranging your garden in a quiet place set back from traffic areas. If the latter, arrange your garden as close to your greenhouse, kitchen, or apothecary as possible for easy access for quick harvests and daily care.

Drainage

Herbs need well-drained soil, so make sure the spot you choose has good drainage. Building raised beds and filling them with good-quality free-draining compost and topsoil will also provide great drainage, allowing excess water to drain through while absorbing the essential moisture and nutrients needed. It is also worth noting that perhaps one of the easiest ways to improve drainage in your garden beds is by growing lots of plants who will absorb the water, thus preventing waterlogging.

Water

Herbs need consistent moisture, so make sure there is a system in place, whether it be drip irrigation, a sprinkler, or water access and a watering can, to water them regularly. Keep the soil damp but not drenched. Overwatering can cause the roots to rot. Generally, as long as you have good drainage, you cannot water too long, just too frequently. In other words, giving your garden one heavy drench first thing in the morning is better than five short showers throughout the day that risk washing away the nutrients in the soil and drowning the roots.

Care

Regular pruning will help keep your herbs healthy and encourage new growth, so harvest daily if you can. Choose a location that will allow you to conveniently visit the garden often to care for it and to harvest.

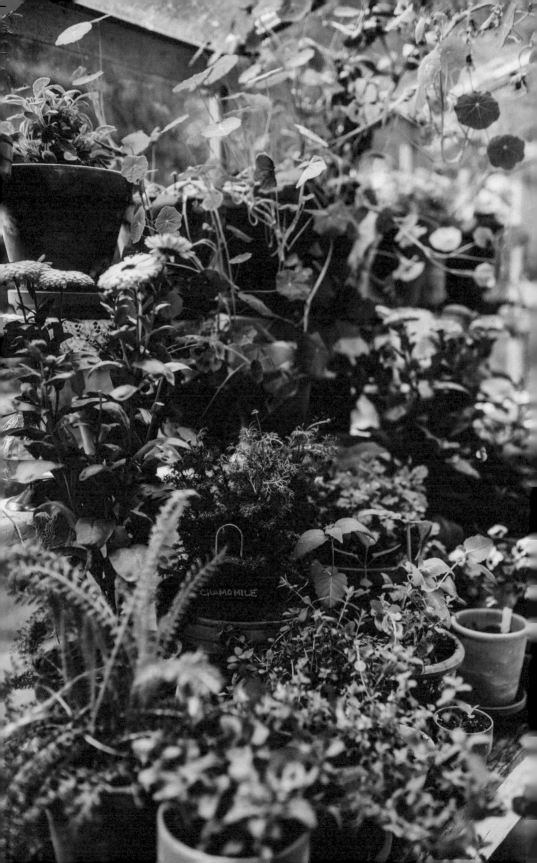

Decisions of an Herb Grower

> "Herbs are the friend of the physician
> and the pride of cooks."
>
> —*Charlemagne* (747–814)

Choosing which herbs to grow in your garden can be both fun and rewarding, but can also be a bit overwhelming at times. Here are some tips to help you make the best decisions and make the most of the garden space available to you.

Consider Needs and Themes

Think about what you want to use the herbs for. Are you looking for culinary herbs to use in your cooking, fragrant long-lasting herbs to add to floral arrangements, beautiful herbs for crafting, or do you want to grow herbs for medicinal purposes and self-care? What herbs do you use most when cooking? What herbal fragrances are your favorites? Answering these questions can help you narrow down your options.

Themed Herb Gardens

One of the many fascinating things about herbs is their natural ability to intermingle with, elevate, and complement other personal interests in your life. Below are nine of my favorite garden themes. Within each theme, I've chosen herbs that are most common but also suitable for someone just beginning to explore and cultivate an herb garden (or garden bed) with that theme. I encourage you to use these lists to further explore herbs that fall into a theme you're interested in or to create themed beds within your existing garden.

Kitchen Herb Garden

Perhaps the most common herb garden theme, kitchen herb gardens (also referred to as culinary herb gardens) are a way to add botanical beauty, color, and flavor to your favorite dishes and culinary experiences. Add flavor to your cuisine with these twelve herbs:

- Basil
- Chive
- Cilantro
- Dill
- Fennel[1]
- Marjoram
- Mints
- Oregano
- Parsley
- Rosemary
- Sage
- Thyme

Cocktail Herb Garden

My favorite way to use herbs is to shake, muddle, or garnish botanical cocktails with them. They add incredible texture, pops of color, and interesting and sometimes delightfully unexpected flavors to your favorite cocktails, mocktails, lemonades, iced waters, and more! Incorporating herbs into drinks served at your next social gathering is sure to bring smiles to the faces of your guests and spark conversations. Here are my go-to herbs for botanically mixed drinks:

- Basil
- Bee balm
- Borage
- Butterfly pea
- Calendula
- Chive
- Fennel[2]
- Lavender
- Lemon balm
- Marigold
- Marjoram
- Mints
- Nasturtium
- Sage
- Thyme
- Viola

Bee & Butterfly Herb Garden

If, like me, you find great joy in watching butterflies flutter around as you read in your garden or are soothed by the slow, rhythmic hum of busy working bees, then the bee and butterfly herb garden (commonly

---

1 Fennel is not the friendliest herbal companion and is best grown in its own container away from most other herbs, especially dill.

2 Fennel is not the friendliest herbal companion and is best grown in its own container away from most other herbs, especially dill.

referred to as a pollinator garden) is for you! While nearly all herbs attract pollinators, I've chosen eighteen below that are particularly bee and butterfly friendly:

- Anise hyssop
- Bee balm
- Borage
- Butterfly pea
- Calendula
- Catnip

- Chive
- Echinacea
- Lavender
- Lemon balm
- Marjoram
- Milkweed

- Mints
- Nasturtium
- Oregano
- Rosemary
- Sage
- Thyme

Natural Dyer's Herb Garden

While not typically the primary function of these botanicals, you may be surprised to learn that all sixteen of the herbs listed below have another superpower: the ability to naturally dye fiber. (We also use the natural dyes created by these herbs as natural watercolors.) A part of (or sometimes the entire) plant will need to be decocted in water to extract the natural dye, a relatively simple process that requires a bit of research, but is well worth it for the experience and gorgeous end product. It is important to note that certain parts of an herb may create different colors. For example, echinacea petals create a purple dye and its leaves create a green dye.

- Butterfly pea
- Calendula
- Chamomile
- Echinacea
- Goldenrod
- Indigo

- Lady's mantle
- Marigold
- Nasturtium
- Nettle
- Pokeberry
- Rosemary

- Saffron
- Sage
- St. John's wort
- Turmeric
- Yarrow

33

A little background on how this theme came to be part of my own backyard garden: in addition to growing herbs and flowers, Cedar House Farm is home to four adorable Southdown babydoll sheep. Some of the herbs in my garden are grown and preserved specifically to naturally dye the wool from our sheep. To bring the sustainability cycle full circle, sheep dung (pelleted droppings) is an excellent organic waste for fertilizing plants and is one of the primary ingredients in our compost blend. The compost is then used as a natural supplement in our garden beds. So, the sheep fertilize my herbs and flowers, which are then used to dye their wool!

Healing Herb Garden

Popular since the Middle Ages, a healing garden has many other common names, including medicinal garden, apothecary garden, and garden of simples. It consists of a collection of herbs that have therapeutic purposes and are used to support different ailments. I've chosen fifteen that I believe are the most widely appreciated or have the largest number of beneficial properties:

- Bee balm
- Calendula
- Catnip
- Chamomile
- Echinacea
- Eucalyptus[3]
- Feverfew
- Ginger
- Holy basil
- Lavender
- Lemon balm
- Oregano
- Peppermint
- Rosemary
- Yarrow

Teatime Herb Garden

Whether iced or hot, tea is the second most consumed drink in the world, after water, and every tea is derived from a plant. If a quiet evening at home or with friends sipping a warm (or iced) herbal beverage is more your *cup of tea* (see what I did there?), then these twenty herbs, which can be used individually or together to create lovely herbal blends, will be the perfect starting point for your teatime herb garden:

- Anise hyssop
- Bee balm
- Borage
- Calendula
- Catnip
- Chamomile
- Echinacea
- Fennel
- Ginger
- Hibiscus
- Holy basil
- Lavender
- Lemon balm
- Lemongrass
- Lilac
- Mints
- Rose
- Rosemary
- Sage
- St. John's wort

---

3 Eucalyptus roots release a toxic chemical that inhibits the growth of any plants growing around it, so keep this in mind when planning your garden beds and provide eucalyptus its own container.

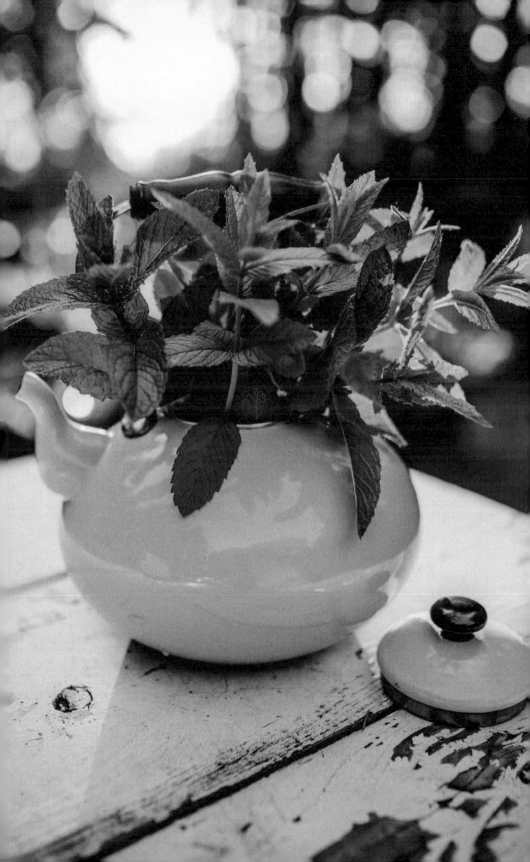

Edimental Herb Garden

A term coined by Stephan Barstow, an edible plant collector and author of *Around the World In 80 Plants*, *edimental* refers to ornamental plants that are also edible. With this as the theme, I've narrowed the playing field a bit more, including the following list of herbs that are both beautiful and edible! Honestly, this was the hardest list for me to create because I see beauty in every edible herb, but here are the eighteen I feel have the most attractive physical characteristics:

- Allium
- Basil
- Bee balm
- Borage
- Butterfly pea
- Calendula
- Chamomile
- Echinacea
- Ginger
- Lavender
- Marigold
- Marjoram
- Mints
- Nasturtium
- Rose
- Safron
- Sage
- Yarrow

Shakespearean Herb Garden

Best known as a playwright, poet and actor, William Shakespeare brought love and loss, passion and tragedy, humor, and wit to the world through his art. Today, gardens worldwide honor his legacy by cultivating a combination of botanicals that were mentioned in his most famous poems and plays. If a passionate, beautiful Elizabethan Garden calls to you, here are fourteen herbs from the quill of Shakespeare all those years ago:

- Anise hyssop
- Chamomile
- Fennel
- Lavender
- Lemon balm
- Marigold
- Marjoram
- Mints
- Parsley
- Rosemary
- Spearmint
- Sweet violet
- Thyme
- Winter savory

Relaxation Herb Garden

If a little rest and relaxation is your idea of a perfect day, perhaps an herb garden dedicated to growing herbs for self-care products is more your vibe. While kava, passionflower, and valerian are the three herbs most researched and recognized for their calming properties, they are not readily available to many of us, so I've chosen to list herbs that are more recognizable and obtainable, as well as valued for their calming, relaxing properties. These fourteen herbs are often found in bath soaks and salts, hot teas, massage oils, salves, balms, soaps, and lotions, among other forms of aromatherapy and self-care products.

- Basil
- California poppy
- Catnip
- Chamomile
- Eucalyptus[4]
- Holy basil (tulsi)
- Hops
- Marjoram
- Lavender
- Lemon balm
- Peppermint
- Rose
- Rosemary
- St. John's wort

Know Your Zone

Different herbs thrive in different environments, so it's important to choose herbs that are well-suited to your climate. Some herbs, like rosemary and thyme, prefer drier, sunnier conditions, while others, like mint and parsley, prefer more shade and moisture. For United States residents, the US Department of Agriculture is a fantastic online resource and has plant hardiness zone maps to take the guesswork out of this process. If, like me, you live in the Pacific Northwest, I highly recommend the Tilth Alliance's Maritime Northwest Gardening Guide's planning calendar.

---

4 Eucalyptus roots release a toxic chemical that inhibits the growth of any plants growing around it, so keep this in mind when planning your garden beds and provide eucalyptus its own container.

Consider Growing Space

Consider the amount of space you have available to grow a garden. Some herbs, like basil and oregano, can grow quite large, while others, like chive and cilantro, stay relatively compact. Some herbs, like mint and nasturtium, grow best in containers or boxes due to their invasive tendencies, while herbs like borage and yarrow would do fine being planted directly in the ground. Keep in mind that you don't need acreage to grow an herb garden. If you have limited space, consider vertical and container gardening. One of the benefits of container gardening is that once the growing season is complete, you can simply pick your containers up and move them indoors to continue to enjoy your herbs year-round.

Understand Your Herbs

Once you have a general idea of which herbs you would like to grow, take the time to research the amount of space they require, care requirements, and uses. Part III of this book is an excellent jumping-off point for determining which herbs are the best fit for you and your garden.

Lifespan

All plants, including herbs, fall into one of three categories distinguished by their lifespan and growing tendencies.

Let's begin with the most common category: annuals. Annual herbs are planted as seeds, emerge in the spring, and die back permanently in autumn, completing their lifestyle in one year. They typically germinate more quickly, grow more quickly, and bloom profusely until they go to seed. Their life cycle ends unless you save their seeds. The beauty of annual herbs is that they tend to have more vibrant colors, attracting the most pollinators. Additionally, some annuals tend to self-sow, meaning they drop seeds in the fall that sprout the following spring in the same location as last year's plant, so they are often confused with perennials. Hearty annuals are more tolerant of cold temperatures (can typically withstand a frost) and can be direct-sown outside. Tender annuals are just as sensitive as they sound and quite intolerant of cold temperatures. They should be started indoors and need warm soil and warm temperatures to survive. Half-hardy annuals fall somewhere in between, perhaps tolerating a very light frost but preferring warmer temps and being started indoors.

Perennial herbs, on the other hand, are initially planted as seeds but return year after year, often for decades, offering long-lasting beauty to your garden or landscape. They tend to be slower and more difficult to germinate, have a slower growth rate, and go dormant during the winter months, emerging stronger the following spring. Perennials are cost-effective, and require less work in the long run, often needing little more than an annual trim, a good weeding every now and again, and, of course, regular watering and harvesting. Because perennials stay in one place permanently, they tend to have a deeper root system, which means they need less watering. Moreover, the deep roots of perennials pull essential nutrients from the soil closer to the surface, indirectly benefiting your annuals and biennials by giving them access to those nutrients. And because they do not require disruption to the soil, the soil around perennials improves over time. If you provide them with the space and quality soil they need, perennials will reemerge every spring bigger and better than the year before.

There is also a less-common third category of herbs, called biennials, which do not produce seeds their first year. Instead, they die back after their first year and then reemerge in the spring, flower, and produce seed, reaching their reproductive stage before dying back permanently. California poppy, clary sage, dill, fennel, mullein, and parsley fall into this category. It is also worth noting that biennials often readily self-seed, making them a permanent fixture in your garden bed, and often are mistakenly branded as perennials.

Annual Herbs for Every Garden:

- Anise hyssop (often self-sows)
- Arugula
- Basil
- Borage
- Calendula
- California poppy
- Chamomile (all but Roman, often self-sows)
- Chervil
- Cilantro/coriander
- Lemon verbena
- Marigold
- Nasturtium
- Summer savory

Perennial Herbs for Every Garden:

- Allium
- Bay laurel
- Bee balm
- Catnip
- Chamomile, Roman[5]
- Chive
- Dill
- Echinacea
- Eucalyptus
- Fennel[6]
- Feverfew
- Ginger
- Holy basil (tulsi)
- Hyssop
- Lavender
- Lemon balm
- Marjoram
- Meadow sweet
- Milkweed
- Mints
- Oregano
- Parsley[7]
- Rose
- Rosemary
- Saffron
- Sage
- St. John's wort
- Thyme
- Winter savory
- Yarrow

Note: Depending on the climate you live in, some herbs may be perennials for you but behave as annuals in a different climate. This list encompasses how the herbs are most commonly portrayed.

I encourage you to consider incorporating a combination of annuals *and* perennials into your herb garden to add seasonal variety and continuous harvests.

---

5 Unlike German and Zloty Lan varieties, Roman Chamomile is actually a perennial!

6 Fennel is considered a short-lived perennial, meaning they live three to five years and then begin to decline.

7 While parsley is technically a biennial (living for only two years), it readily self-seeds, making it a permanent fixture in your garden bed.

Choose Organic

Choose organic herb seeds and starters to avoid exposure to chemicals and pesticides that may have negative impacts on your health. Additionally, because organic farming practices prioritize soil health, studies have shown that organic plants are stronger and have higher nutrient content.

Experiment

Don't be afraid to grow new herbs and experiment with different varieties. I hope that the following pages not only reinforce your interest in growing herbs, but also introduce you to new varieties of herbs that may be a wonderful fit for you. Growing herbs is a fun and rewarding experience, and you never know what you will discover along the way!

Garden Dreaming

One of my favorite things to do during the darkest days of winter is plan my summer garden. I begin by mapping out the growing space available to me using a dot grid notebook that will become my gardening journal for the year, my blank botanical canvas. Garden planning is a promise of something more to come. An act of preparation for a new season. A vision of what will be. A reflection of who I am. Before I purchase seeds, I take time to draw out my garden beds and containers, indicating where the best light is, any structures or trees that may obstruct or dapple the light throughout the day, and what type of light each bed or container receives throughout the growing season. Sectioning off each bed into "full sun," "partial shade," and "full shade" helps me determine where each plant should go. Then, I draw in any perennials that currently exist in the beds and containers.

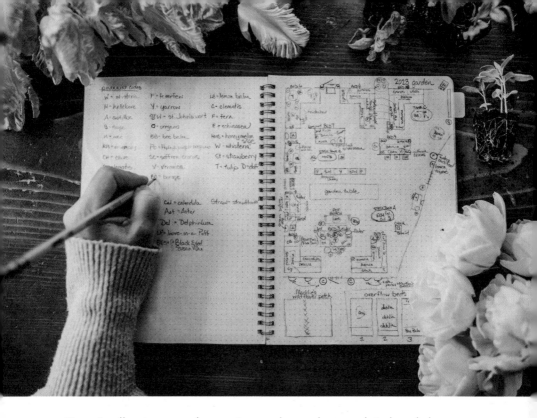

Next, I pull out my seed organizer and see what seeds I already have, and which of them I want to grow. Lastly, I make a wish list of all the perennials and annuals I hope to grow this year and begin to place them in the garden map. Don't be afraid to make a mood board, draw or watercolor details into your maps, or make lists upon lists of all the ideas and inspiration you have for your growing space.

Once you have a plan, you're ready to buy seeds! My favorite herb seed suppliers are Baker Creek Heirloom Seeds Company, Johnny's Selected Seeds, Floret Flowers, Uprising Organic Seeds, and Strictly Medicinal Seeds. It is thanks to these five incredible seed suppliers that my personal seed inventory has become a well-crafted and curated collection that I'm very proud of. I also sell a small batch of seeds saved from my own backyard garden each year and have them available in my shop. Brace yourself, though—seed shopping is addicting!

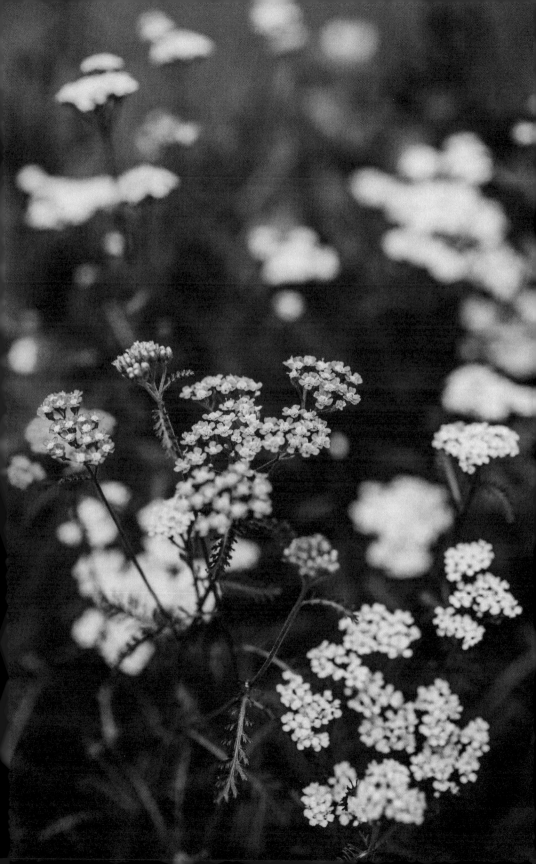

"How doth the little busy bee
Improve each shining hour,
And gather honey all the day
From every opening flower!"

—*Isaac Watts*, English poet and
Congregationalist minister (1674–1748)

Creating a Pollinator Haven

When you grow a pollinator-friendly garden with herbs, no matter how big or small, you create a vital ecosystem that supports a variety of plant and animal life. Pollinators like bees, butterflies, and hummingbirds are responsible for pollinating many of the fruits, vegetables, and flowers that we enjoy. Without them, our food supply and natural beauty would be greatly diminished. By planting herbs and other fragrant and colorful plants and flowers, and providing habitat for these important creatures, we make a positive impact on our world, and help ensure a healthy and thriving ecosystem for ourselves and future generations.

My garden is filled with colorful and fragrant flowers and herbs that attract and feed birds and other pollinators such as honeybees, native bees, moths, and butterflies. When I harvest, I make sure to always leave plenty behind to keep them busy and happy. It brings me so much joy to attract life and buzzing around me as I work in my garden. To hear the beautiful birdsong. To watch my neighbor's honeybees make their daily rounds through my garden beds collecting nectar, or a pair of butterflies as they flutter by in their cyclone formation, oblivious to my gaze. We even have a resident hummingbird who has taken ownership over the garden space and his hanging feeder, quickly running off any other birds that attempt to visit. And then there are the chickadees—perhaps my favorite of all the peaceful sounds I hear while I'm tending to my garden beds, with their fluty birdsong that has the ability to lift my spirits no matter how drained I may feel. Thanks to so many herbs, my garden hums with life from dawn to dusk like never before, attracting family, friends, and pollinators alike, and inviting them in to stay a while.

How Do You Know if a Plant Is Pollinator Friendly?

A plant listed as pollinator friendly typically means it is rich in nectar and pollen for insects and that the shape and color of the flower encourages pollinators to visit. Pollinator-friendly plants often have trumpet-shaped or open-center blooms, or flower heads that are easy for pollinators to land on and crawl across. Pollinator-friendly plants are also typically brightly colored to attract our busy friends and are always free of chemicals and pesticides.

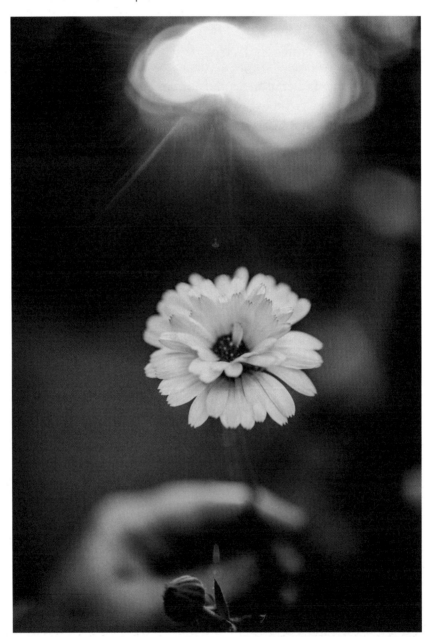

Tips for Creating a Beautiful and Thriving Pollinator Garden

- Plant lots of flowers and herbs in a location that gets at least six hours of sun daily.

- Plant flowering herbs that bloom at different times to attract pollinators on an ongoing basis.

- Plant large groupings of the same plant. These "pollinator targets" are more easily spotted from the air.

- Grow several varieties of flowers and herbs of different shapes, colors, and fragrances to attract as many species of insects and birds as possible. Honeybees are most drawn to yellow, white, and blue, while moths prefer white or gray fragrant plants, similar to what you might see in a moon garden.

- Grow herbs with lovely fragrances.

- Grow bushy herbs, such as rosemary, yarrow, and feverfew, that provide pollinators with shelter from the elements.

- Provide a water source for pollinators, such as a shallow bowl of water or a birdbath.

- Eliminate all use of chemicals and pesticides. Keep in mind that most pollinators are beneficial insects that will help you control pests. For example, ladybugs feast on aphids.

- When collecting seeds in autumn, leave some for the birds to snack on over the winter months. Dead flower heads also provide shelter to beneficial insects during the coldest months.

To Sow Seeds or Plant Starts

It's time, friend. Time to get our hands dirty. There's something so soothing about working with soil. The smell, the texture, the idea of caring for a plant that will provide health benefits for your entire family. Spring is for laying the foundation for a bountiful summer harvest. For sowing the seeds for a slower life. For taking time to appreciate the longer days and waking hours it offers. I've found that gardening improves my mood when I'm having a difficult day and gives me a feeling of peacefulness and contentment. My hope is that you, too, will experience similar mental health benefits when working in your herb garden. Let the soil sift through your fingers. Take the time to learn about what you're growing. Enjoy and appreciate each step of the process.

Benefits of Growing from Seed

> "What made it her garden was the way she could look at a handful of tiny seeds in the bareness of winter and imagine how they could be, months later, sunlit and in flower. It was as if she painted with blooms."
>
> —*Geraldine Brooks*, Year of Wonders

Growing herbs from seed is a rewarding experience with many benefits. It is an opportunity to nourish yourself mentally and can be mood-lifting during those last dark weeks of winter, which gives this method a leg up over purchasing starter plants later in the year.

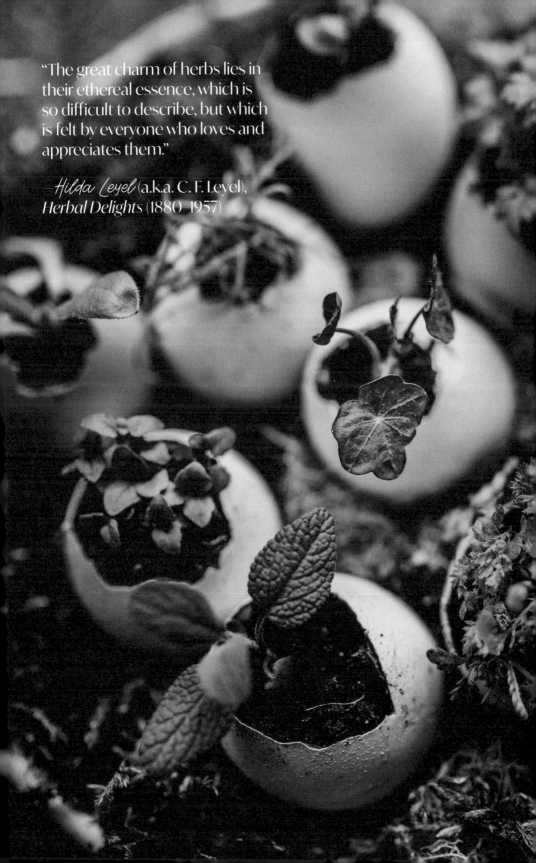

"The great charm of herbs lies in their ethereal essence, which is so difficult to describe, but which is felt by everyone who loves and appreciates them."

Hilda Leyel (a.k.a. C. F. Leyel), *Herbal Delights* (1880–1957)

Here are just a few reasons why starting your herbs from seed is a great choice:

Selection

When you grow herbs from seed, you have access to a much wider variety of plant options. Nurseries and garden centers may have a limited selection of varieties, but when buying seeds, you can choose from dozens of different varieties within a single type of herb, each with their unique flavors, fragrances, and physical properties. Growing from seed opens an entirely new world of possibilities to your garden.

Cost

Growing herbs from seed is much more cost-effective than purchasing starter plants. While a packet of seeds may cost a few dollars, there are usually anywhere from 8-50 seeds in a single packet, whereas a single starter plant can cost several times more.

Quality Control

When you start your own herbs from seed, you have sole control over the quality of your plants. You control what is in the soil, what types of fertilizers are used, and you can select the healthiest, strongest seedlings to transplant into your garden, which can result in stronger, more resilient plants that are better able to resist disease and pests.

Robustness

Generally speaking, plants grown organically from seed produce a more robust root structure than those grown from cuttings or with the use of chemicals. Seed-grown plants are stronger, more resilient, have a better yield, and last longer.

Experience

Starting herbs from seed can be an educational and rewarding experience for gardeners of all ages. There's something deeply satisfying about growing your own plants from seed. Watching tiny seeds sprout into thriving plants is a fulfilling experience that can provide a sense of accomplishment and pride and every growing season brings with it opportunities to observe, learn, and problem solve. It's also a great way to teach children about the life cycle of plants and gain hands-on experience in caring for even the tiniest seedlings.

Benefits of Choosing Starter Plants

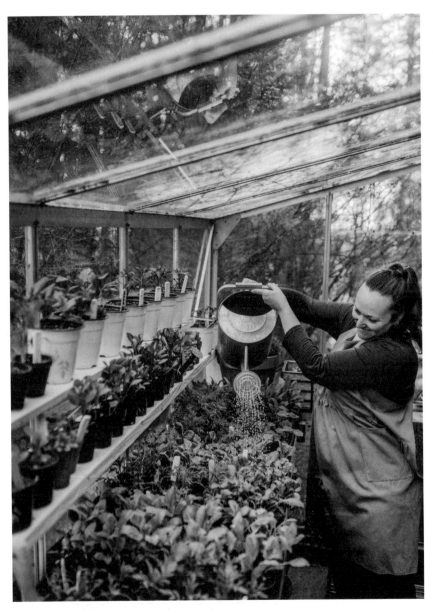

"He who plants a garden plants happiness."

—Chinese Proverb

Growing from seed requires time and patience and is not ideal for everyone. Here are several benefits to buying starter herb plants instead of growing them from seed:

Convenience

Buying starter plants is a more convenient option for those who don't have the time or space to start their own seeds. Starter plants are already well-established and can be transplanted directly into the garden or container, saving time and effort.

Greater Certainty

When buying starter plants, you have a greater degree of certainty about what you're getting. You can see the plant and assess its health and size before purchasing it, ensuring it is healthy and viable. To assess, check that the foliage and stems are green (not wilted or yellow) and there are no signs of disease, or pest damage. If you notice that the starter plant seems to be missing a lot of its leaves, pass on that plant. It is likely diseased, and the yellowed or pest-damaged leaves were removed but the pests or disease may remain. Check the root system for healthy, white roots that are evenly distributed throughout the soil by gently loosening and lifting the plant out of the container.

Expedited Results

Starter plants are simply further along in their growth process than seeds, which means you can enjoy fresh herbs sooner. This can be particularly beneficial if you're starting your herb garden later in the season.

Beginner Gardener-Friendly

Starting plants from seed can be quite challenging for beginners. Starter plants, on the other hand, offer a more straightforward way to get started with herb gardening, without having to worry about germinating seeds and providing the proper growing conditions.

Higher Success Rate

Starting plants from seed can be unpredictable, with some seeds failing to germinate or producing weak seedlings. Buying starter plants can increase your chances of success, as you're starting with a more established, healthy plant.

Earth and Seed

Direct Sowing

Direct sowing is a popular method of planting seeds directly into the ground rather than starting them indoors and transplanting them out later into their permanent homes. It has many advantages. Because there is less preparation, it is considerably more efficient, simpler, eco-friendlier, and less costly. Additionally, there is no hardening off process needed as seedlings that were started outside tend to be more robust.

Sowing directly into the ground has its share of disadvantages as well. Germination takes longer with direct sown seeds, without the luxury of a heat mat to expedite the process, or due to uncontrollable external factors such as unfavorable weather or harsh temperatures. You will sow more seeds than will germinate when you direct sow, which can become costly and inconvenient if garden space is at a premium. Because you must wait to sow them until all threat of frost has passed, direct sown seeds become established plants much later, shortening your growing season. Directly sown seedlings are also more vulnerable to garden pests such as slugs.

Here are a few tips when direct sowing seeds to help ensure that your seeds have the best chance of germinating and growing into healthy, productive herb plants.

53

Timing

Direct sowing seeds should be done when the soil temperature and weather conditions are appropriate for the seeds you are planting, typically after all threat of frost has passed and soil can be worked. It is important to get this right, so check the back of your seed packet (or seed supplier's website) for information on the best time to direct sow each type of seed.

Bed Preparation

Before sowing seeds, prepare their growing area by amending the soil and removing weeds, rocks, and debris. Loosen the soil to a depth of six to eight inches and add compost or other organic matter to improve soil fertility. (For more information on soil health and testing, see "Soil" on page 71.)

Watering

Keep the soil consistently moist after sowing seeds, but avoid over-watering, which can lead to rotting or disease. A light watering with a watering can or spray bottle is often sufficient.

Protection

Protect herb seeds from birds, rodents, and other pests by covering the planting area with netting or using row covers or plastic domes. Remove covers once the seeds have germinated.

Watch the Weather

If you are direct sowing, keep a close eye on overnight temperatures during early spring. While the last frost date for each zone is typically trustworthy, Mother Nature can be quite unpredictable at times. If overnight temperatures fall close to freezing or snow is possible, I drop a plastic dome or row cover over any seedlings that are exposed, to protect them.

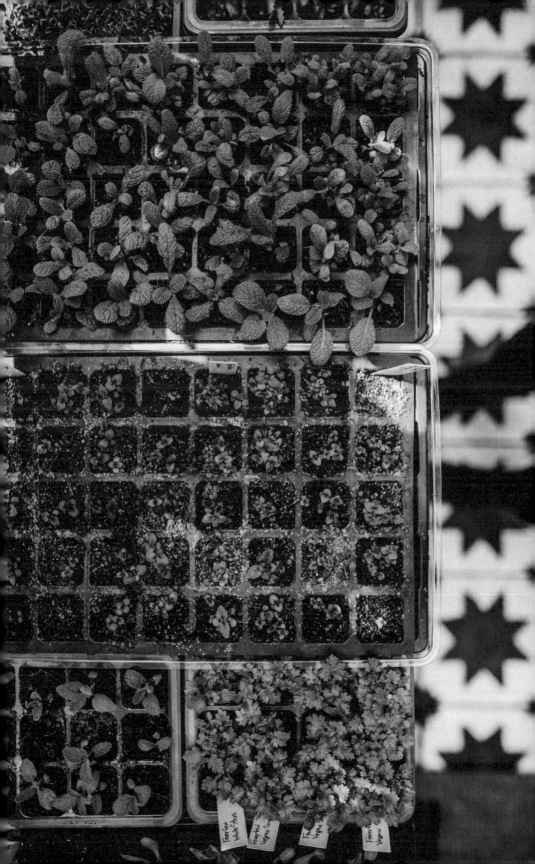

Starting Seeds Indoors

"The love of gardening is a seed once
sown that never dies."

—*Gertrude Jekyll*, British horticulturalist
and garden designer (1843-1932)

Herb Grower's Toolkit

- organic herb seeds of choice
- seed trays, cell trays with drainage holes and plastic domes, or other pots with drainage holes
- organic potting soil (or see my soil recipe below)
- trowel
- large bowl (if using my soil recipe)
- label tags and permanent marker pen
- vermiculite
- heat mat
- grow lights
- water mister
- narrow spout watering can

After a long winter, I'm always grateful to finally have my hands in soil again, sowing big dreams that start with the tiniest of seeds. There is truly nothing like the thrill of seeing those first seedlings emerge; a promise of a new gardening season to come. The greenhouse is my winter sanctuary. And at the heart of it all is the potting bench my husband made me with scraps of wood from around our property. It's where thousands of seeds have germinated under my carefully watching eye. Where my soil-stained hands potted up seedlings and documented grow-along projects. It's where many dreams were sown.

With regard to herbs, it is worth noting that herbs can be a bit more finicky to germinate and maintain than most flowers and vegetables. This is because, historically, herbs have simply been cultivated on a much smaller scale and by fewer people. They often have longer germination windows and more complex growing processes. With this in mind, here are some tips for getting a head start on your gardening season by starting herb seeds indoors:

Containers

Use clean, sterile containers that are at least two inches deep with drainage holes. You can use ceramic, plastic, or biodegradable pots, soil blocking, egg containers, or seed trays. I encourage you to try different containers to choose the ones that work best for you. It's important to consider the root systems of the herbs you're growing and what kind of room they require. Transplant your seedlings into larger pots when you see roots protruding through your drainage holes or if the plants appear to be struggling or stunted in growth. If using old pots or previously used seed trays, be sure to wash them with a bleach water solution (a one-to-ten ratio of bleach to water) to get rid of anything lingering that could cause havoc on your new growing journey.

Purchasing new seed-starting cells, trays, and domes adds up quickly! As an alternative to purchasing new, here are my five favorite seed-starting DIYs using items you likely have around your home.

Five Ecofriendly Seed-Starting Containers

1. 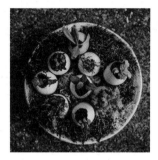 **Eggshells** When cracking eggs to save the shell for this purpose, crack and open the egg on the top quarter of the pointed end of the egg. Empty the egg, fill it with your seed-starting soil mix, and plant your seed as instructed on your seed packet (or in Part III of this book). Before watering, take a knife or garden snips (anything sharp you have handy) and tap on the bottom of the filled eggshell to create a drainage hole in the bottom, being careful not to spill your newly sown contents. Keep the soil evenly moist as your seedlings grow. When you're ready to transplant them to your garden, hold the eggshell in your cupped palm and give it a good squeeze to crack the sides and bottom of the shell. If this proves difficult, use a pair of snips to poke a few holes in the bottom. The inner membrane of the shell will hold your contents in place and save you from a big mess, and the cracks will allow the moisture from your garden bed soil to disintegrate the egg membrane over time as your seedling grows. The best part about this upcycled container is that the eggshell naturally provides your seedling with extra calcium, while simultaneously aerating the soil so your root system can grow and stretch.

2. **Egg Cartons** Cardboard egg cartons are perfectly designed to act as seed-starting trays. They are equipped with individual "cells," and the cardboard material naturally drains excess water and biodegrades over time. Simply take your used cardboard carton, carefully tear off the lid, and fill with your seed-starting mix. If you are sowing seeds that require complete darkness to germinate, leave the lid attached to cover your cells until germination and then tear it off once your sprouts have surfaced. When it's time to plant your seedlings out, the cells can be easily torn apart and planted separately, using the spacing recommended for that herb.

3.

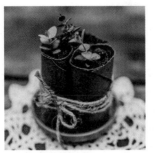

Toilet Paper Rolls I learned this hack early in my gardening career. Toilet paper rolls are a great size (vertical space for your seedlings' new roots to stretch out) and cardboard naturally drains excess water and biodegrades over time. To make, take an empty toilet paper roll (core) and cut one-inch slits evenly around one end. Fold each segment in toward the center, hooking them together to act as the bottom of the cup. Create sets of three or four toilet paper cups and tie them together with twine to stabilize them. Need a tray to collect excess water and keep them standing straight? Cut an empty milk carton two inches above the bottom. It will perfectly fit four toilet-paper-roll cups.

4.

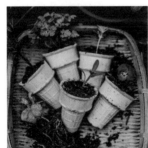

Ice Cream Cones Flat-bottomed ice cream cones are another inexpensive seed-starting container that you might already have around your home. They provide vertical space for your seedlings to develop their root systems, are designed to naturally drain, and you can transplant the entire cone into your garden bed. The cone will biodegrade once it's in the ground, making it another great option for seedlings that resent transplanting.

5.

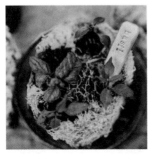

Loofah Sponges You read that right! If you grow your own loofah, you can cut them into three-to-four-inch-tall segments to make perfectly sized, naturally draining, biodegradable cups for holding soil and starting your seeds. Also, do you remember that egg carton lid you tore off your egg carton seed starter container? It will work perfectly to hold your seed-starting loofahs together and collect excess drainage.

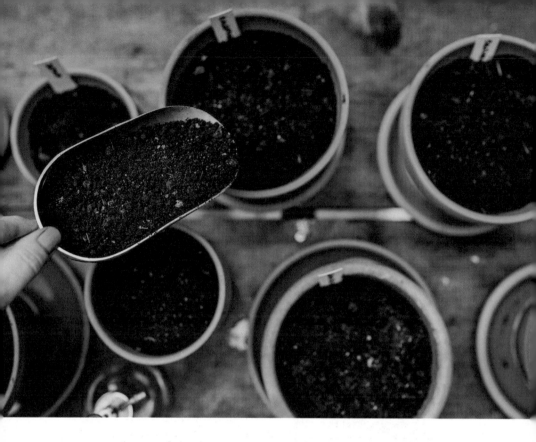

Soil Matters

Use a high-quality organic potting soil that is specifically formulated for seed starting. Avoid using garden soil, which can be heavy and may contain disease-causing pathogens.

Here is my seed-starting soil recipe:

Cedar House Living Seed-Starting Soil Recipe

1 cup of organic soil or compost mixture

1 cup organic coconut coir

3 cups worm castings

½ cup sand

2 tablespoons gypsum

½ cup fireplace ash (biochar) from your bonfire or fireplace (optional)

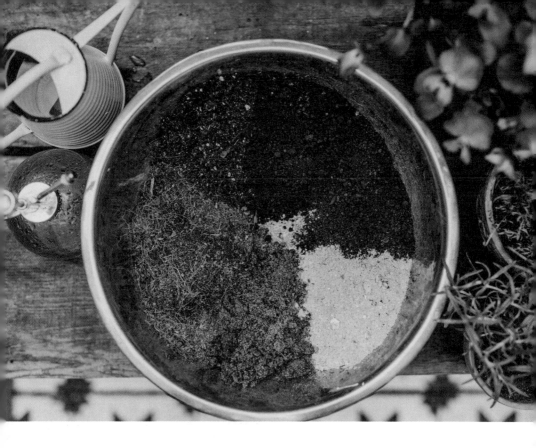

"To forget how to dig the earth
and tend the soil is to forget ourselves."

—*Mahatma Gandhi,* Indian lawyer and
political ethicist (1869–1948)

Combine all the ingredients in a large bowl, mix well, and then add
water, starting with one cup, until the soil mixture holds together
when squeezed in your hand without crumbling. The consistency
should not be soupy or muddy. Then transfer it into your seed-starting
trays, tapping the tray on the table a couple times to remove large
air pockets.

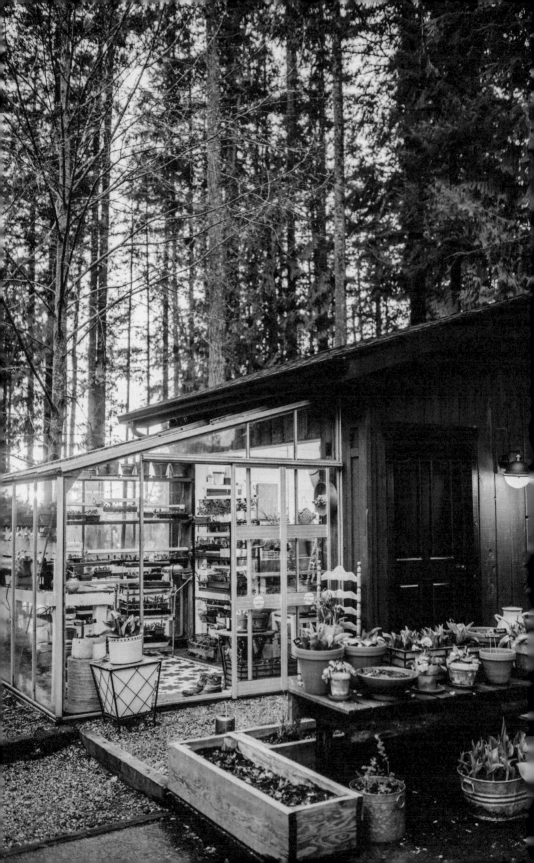

Sowing Seeds

Once your containers or seed trays are filled, double-check the back of your seed packet to confirm that this is the appropriate time to sow these seeds. This will require you to know your zone, so that you can safely determine your frost date and then count back the number of weeks recommended on the seed packet. Sow your seeds, one or two in each cell, or broadcast if recommended (more on broadcasting follows). The seed packet (or supplier's website) should specify if the seed needs light to germinate, or if it requires complete darkness. Seeds with a hard seed coat, like lavender, should be carefully nicked, scratched, or brushed with sandpaper (scarification), while other seeds, like echinacea and marshmallow, require a period of cold conditioning (stratification) to successfully germinate.

If the seeds require light, surface-sow the seed by dropping it on top of the soil and leaving it uncovered. Add a dusting of vermiculite or coconut coir to the top of every seedling tray to ward off algae growth, which is common in the warm, damp growing conditions new seedlings require. Then carefully water the seeds by holding a water mister a full arm's length above the seed tray and letting the mist fall down gently. This technique has worked well for me to prevent the force of the water from pushing tiny seeds (sometimes smaller than a grain of sand) to the side of the tray or blowing them out of the tray altogether.

If your seed requires darkness to germinate, the package will typically indicate that they should be sown into the soil and covered. In most cases, large seeds, such as nasturtium, are best sown quite deeply, and tiny seeds like chamomile are best strewn on the surface. If the package does not specify how deep to sow, I typically only sow it as deep as the thickness of the seed itself. Add a thin layer of vermiculite or coconut coir as the top layer. Carefully water them with the misting bottle (letting the mist fall from above as previously described), add a very thin layer of vermiculite, and label them with the type of herb and variety.

I typically move from a misting bottle to a narrow-spouted watering can once my seedlings have grown two sets of true leaves and developed a taproot system. I am careful to use lukewarm water, instead of cold water directly from the hose or faucet, to prevent the fragile seedlings from going into shock. In fact, I fill my misting bottles and watering cans with water and leave them on my heat mat to keep the water the perfect temperature when I need it. Above all else, when sowing seeds, take time to appreciate the simplicity and timelessness of this activity, and immerse yourself in a practice that is as old as time.

Broadcast Sowing

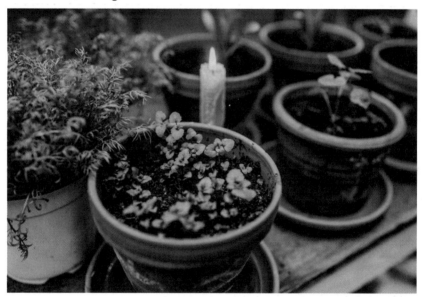

From time to time, I prefer to broadcast sow my seeds (sprinkling them out onto a larger surface, rather than placing an individual seed in a single tray cell). This method is simpler and more efficient than traditional sowing in rows or cells and works well for herbs that don't have large root systems and don't require careful spacing. I broadcast-sow bee balm, chamomile, chive, cilantro, and lemon balm. I love to broadcast-sow into old vintage vessels that I pick up at my local thrift stores and antique shops. Examples of pieces I've used are vintage library card catalog drawers, old chick feeders, galvanized buckets and watering cans, antique metal pots, cast-iron urns, old concrete bird baths, and terracotta pots. I drill some additional drainage holes in the bottom, if needed, then fill the bottom with a layer of pebbles for additional drainage. Next, I fill the rest of the container to the top with my seed-starting soil mixture and give the top layer a healthy water with the misting bottle. Then I sprinkle the seeds across the top of the soil. If the seed packet indicates that the seeds require light to germinate, I carefully mist the seeds with the misting can (using the waterfall method I described in the previous paragraph), add a very light dusting of vermiculite, and I'm done. If the seed packet indicates that the seeds should be buried, I gently rake the top layer of soil with my fingers, mist very gently, and then cover with a sprinkle more of soil and a thin layer of vermiculite. Lastly, I label the pot or tray with the herb and variety.

Light

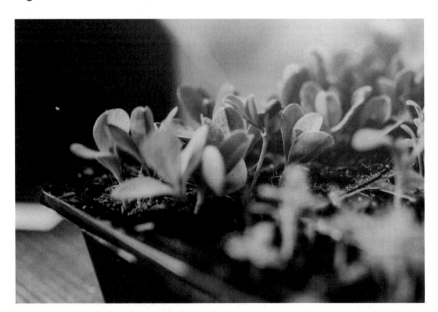

Most herbs require light to germinate, though a few require complete darkness. It's important to read your soil packets or grow guides from seed suppliers to understand how to grow each variety of seed. For seeds that require light to germinate, place containers in a warm, bright location, such as a sunny windowsill or under grow lights. If, like me, you live somewhere that is rather dark in the winter, grow lights are a very important tool for successful germination and can even be used as your sole light source if you are growing in a basement or other room with no windows. Both florescent and LED lights work fine, but I prefer LED. They vary in strength, size, and shape, so you can choose what works best for your growing space, and often also have automatic timers, dimmers, and fans built into the device. Grow lights should be positioned three to five inches above the highest leaf in your seedling tray. If the grow light is too high, your seedlings will "reach" for them and become leggy. If the grow light is too low, it will scorch the leaves, dry out the soil too quickly, and ultimately kill the plant. Pay attention to how each variety of plant is responding to the light source and adjust accordingly. Pay special attention to high-wattage LED lights, as they may need to be placed a couple inches farther away from your seedlings to prevent the leaves from turning a deep red or brown, or scorching the leaves and drying out the soil. Grow lights should be used as a supplement to daylight. In other words, turn the grow lights on in the morning to supplement what sunlight there is during the day, and then turn them off at night so the seedlings can rest and build energy.

As your plants continue to grow taller, adjust grow lights so they are always three to five inches higher than the tops of your plants. If you are growing using only natural light, be mindful that the sun will reposition a bit each day as we move closer to the next solstice. You may find shadows on your plants that were not there the day before. Reposition your plant locations as needed, and add artificial light if your seedlings are not thriving.

Temperature

Nearly all seeds require warmth to germinate. I highly recommend using a seedling heat mat, which typically cuts your germination period by half or more. If you have a friend or neighbor who has a heat mat you can borrow, even better, as you'll only need it for a short period of time. Keep the air temperature around 65–75 degrees Fahrenheit.

> Note: Seedlings should be removed from the heat mat (and plastic dome lids removed) as soon as they have sprouted. Delaying this step can end in long, "leggy" seedlings that will be difficult to maintain and grow. Because this can happen at different times for each type of seed, it is best to sow each variety in separate containers or trays, so you can move one variety of seed off of heat while you are still patiently waiting for another type of seed to germinate.

Soil Moisture

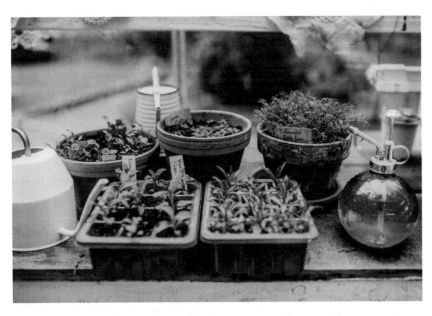

Herb seeds need to be kept moist to germinate, but avoid overwatering, which will quickly cause your seeds to rot. Bottom-water by placing the containers in a tray of water and allowing the soil to absorb the moisture through the drainage holes. Using a heat dome significantly helps retain moisture (and warmth) in tray cells too. If you don't have a dome, plastic wrap will work. After your seeds have sprouted, remove the dome, and use a water mister or spray bottle to keep the top level of soil evenly moist without drowning your tiny new sprouts.

Continue to water your seedlings whenever the soil becomes dry. You can also check the soil moisture level by pushing your finger about a half-inch into the soil. If it feels dry, it's time to water. The size and depth of your container, type of soil you use, and strength of grow and natural light all play a role in how often you will need to water. This could be once a week or every day, depending on the size and depth of the container. I have found that I never need to water my seedlings more than every two to three days when they are small. As a general rule, I'd rather my soil be a tad too dry than too moist. If the seedlings begin to wilt or the edges of their leaves turn brown, don't panic. They will typically perk back up after they've been given a good drink, as long as you didn't ignore their cries for help too long. But once their roots have been drowned, you have to start over from scratch.

Thin Seedlings

It is common to plant more than one seed in each tray cell to best utilize your growing space and increase your likelihood of growing the quantity of seeds you desire from each variety. Once your seeds have sprouted, thin them out (this is sometimes referred to as "pricking out") to one seedling per cell, to prevent overcrowding. This is definitely one of the most difficult tasks for me to do, because I instinctively want to see all my seedlings grow into plants, but it is important to give your seedlings sufficient space to grow and develop properly. If I have a cell where no seed germinated, I also attempt to relocate one of the pricked-out sprouts to that cell. I would estimate that my success rate with transplanting newly emerged seedlings is about 75 percent, so I always try.

Circulation

Air circulation is important to the health of the plant. If you are growing in a lived-in space of your home (kitchen window, living room bay, etc.) then you likely have plenty of circulation in the space already. But if you are growing in a basement, greenhouse, or covered porch that doesn't have as much walk-through traffic or heat registers, consider adding a small fan to circulate air throughout the day. Also, brushing your hand lightly back and forth over the top of your seedlings every now and then (almost like you are petting them) will help them to become stockier and stronger.

Nutrients

Once your plant has a few sets of true leaves (these are the leaves that grow *after* the first set of cotyledon leaves), it is time to supplement your plant's diet. It is critical that you only use organic supplements on your herbs. I use Neptune Harvest Organic Fish & Seaweed Fertilizer and AgroThrive All Purpose Organic Liquid Fertilizer. Fertilizers are important to add micronutrients to your soil and strengthen the root systems of your plants. When fertilizing young seedlings, I recommend diluting the recommended indoor plant package instructions by 50 percent. For example, if the package instructions recommend one tablespoon of fertilizer for one gallon of water, use half a tablespoon. Do this until the plants are six inches tall, then use the fertilizer doses recommended on the package. When fertilizing your herbs, remember that you want to fertilize the root system, not the stem, leaves, and blooms, so try to water around your plant rather than over the top of it. Because you will harvest the aerial parts of the plant (leaves and flowers), I recommend spraying the leaves with a round of fresh water afterward, to rinse them of any fertilizer drops that may have settled on them during application. Lastly, but very importantly, do not overfertilize. Dilute the dosage as instructed, and only fertilize small plants every few weeks.

69

Potting Up

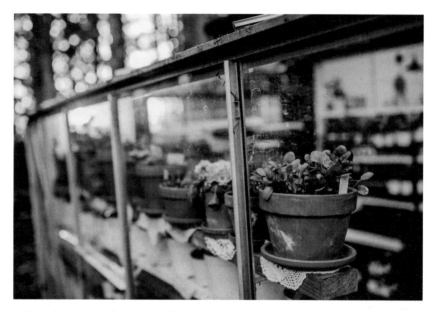

When the roots of your seedling begin to poke through the drainage hole at the bottom of the seed trays, it is time to pot them up. "Potting up" simply refers to the process of transplanting seedlings from their original seed tray containers into larger containers that have more room for the plant and root system to continue to grow and develop. To pot up your seedlings, take your larger pot and fill the bottom of it with a high-quality organic compost. Then carefully pinch the bottom of the seedling tray to loosen the seedling from the walls of the tray and tip it out into your hand. Carefully loosen the root system on the bottom and place it in the new pot. Fill around the plant with compost and give it a good drink of water. Seedlings that have been potted up will have access to more soil, which means more nutrients, leading to stronger, healthier plants. Potting up often means you will have to water less, *but* it can be a lengthy process depending on how many seedlings you are growing, and you will have to reevaluate the amount of space you have under your grow lights to make sure you can accommodate the larger containers. If you time it right, you may be able to plant your seedlings out directly from their original seed trays, which is ideal.

Garden-Bound

"The earth says much to those who listen."

—*Rumi*, Afghan philosopher (1207–1273)

Soil

Happy soil below ground leads to happy plants above. In the gardening world there is a golden rule that states that the better your soil, the better your harvests. Good-quality soil is alive and made up of organic matter, air, microorganisms, water, and mineral particles. The soil should be loose to allow for air circulation, good drainage, and root growth. To create a healthy bed of soil, fill your beds and containers with a soil rich in humus, plus organic material such as aged manure, plant debris, and compost that continues to break down and naturally fertilize your garden over time. Organic matter helps maintain a neutral pH and will improve the structure of all types of soil. If you find that your soil is heavy and mostly clay, adding organic matter will loosen it. If you find that your soil is too light and sandy, causing water to drain through too quickly before the roots can absorb it for nourishment, adding organic matter can balance it by helping to hold the soil together to retain more moisture. Lastly, organic matter, specifically compost, feeds the earthworms (and microbial life) in your soil that tunnel through and provide natural aeration and draining while simultaneously leaving castings that increase the soil's fertility.

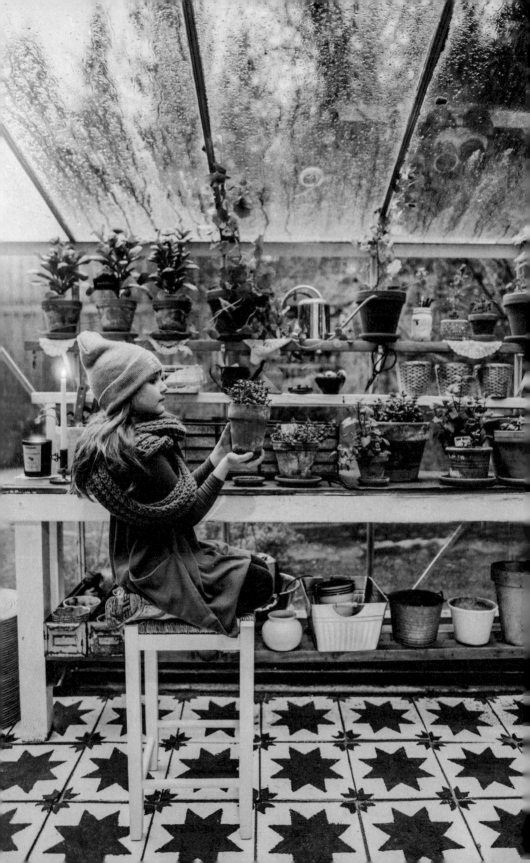

If you are starting with an existing bed of soil, one option is to conduct a simple soil test. Soil testing kits are sold online or can be obtained locally at your local hardware store or nursery. A basic soil test will give you readings for the pH (herbs generally like acidic to neutral soil with a pH in the 6–7 range), phosphorus (P), potassium (K), calcium (Ca), sulfur (S), and magnesium (Mg) currently present in your soil and can provide recommendations for how to adjust these levels if necessary. Understanding what nutrients your soil is missing is the first step. From here, you want to add organic amendments as needed. For example, worm castings are an excellent amendment for soil low in nitrogen, and bone meal is a great option for soil low in phosphorus and/or calcium. More often than not, these tests simply suggest that a regular dose of fertilizer and fresh compost will do the trick.

Would you believe me if I told you I've never performed a soil test on my garden beds? It's true. As an alternative to soil testing, you can do what I did and simply familiarize yourself with the soil. Take the time to observe and understand it and it will, in most cases, tell you everything you need to know. I evaluate my soil annually by asking these five questions:

73

What does it feel like? *When you hold healthy soil in your hands, it will feel a bit loose, cool, and damp, and will crumble relatively easily. It should not be dusty or too dry, extremely sandy, or dripping wet. It should not be too compacted.*

What does it smell like? *Fertile soil smells musty and earthy, due to the beneficial microbes present in it. It should not smell sour, metallic, or like ammonia.*

What does it look like? *Healthy soil is dark brown or near black in color. Dark color is a sign of decomposed organic matter, earthworm activity, aeration, and good drainage. Soil in poor condition will be pale brown or even gray-looking.*

What does it sound like? *When you cut a spade or hand trowel into your soil, what do you hear? Healthy soil will make a smooth,* slightly gritty sound and your spade will go all the way in without too much trouble. If you hear a clink and your spade halts, you most likely have rocky soil, which will need to be addressed. If you hear very gritty, raspy sounds, your soil is likely very sandy and loamy. And a very smooth, sticky sound means your soil is primarily clay.

What does it taste like? Gotcha! Just kidding. I don't taste-test my soil and you shouldn't either.

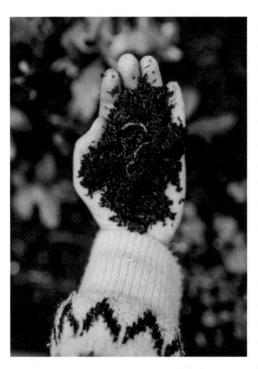

Is there earthworm activity? Earthworms are a sign of healthy soil. If you see them, thank them for the work they're doing. They aerate your soil by burrowing and creating tunnel systems and channels that allow for better air circulation and improved drainage. Earthworms also supplement the soil by digesting organic matter and excreting it in the form of castings that are rich in nutrients and improve the overall soil structure. They also help cycle nutrients through the soil, consuming organic matter and then converting it into nutrients that are then available to your plants. Keep in mind that earthworms require a suitable environment to thrive, so if they are present and happy, it is a sure sign of healthy soil and a healthy ecosystem. Soil with no earthworms is likely contaminated or deficient.

There are a few things you can do to attract earthworms to your garden. First, mix plenty of organic compost into the top layer of your garden beds. Earthworms particularly enjoy decaying organic matter, but any compost available to you will help draw them in. Additionally, refrain from tilling the soil. In time, this "no-till" soil management method will significantly improve the texture and structure of the soil, making it rich and healthy, a perfect home for earthworms. If that still doesn't bring all the worms inching to the yard, try adding a thick layer of mulch. Not only will mulching help suppress weeds, but it also retains moisture around your plant base, and the cool dampness underneath is the perfect earthworm habitat. Lastly, always refrain from using chemicals or pesticides in your garden, which will contaminate your herbs and kill your earthworms. And if all that still doesn't do the trick, you can often find bags of earthworms sold by the pound at your local garden centers, farm stores, or bait shops. Simply sprinkle them evenly throughout your garden beds.

Pull the Competition

Weeding is quite possibly one of the most important tasks you can do to maintain your herb garden. Falling behind on this task can become overwhelming and intimidating very quickly. Weeds come out of nowhere, it often seems, taking over garden space rapidly, and stunting your beautiful herbs by competing for the resources (water, nutrients, even sunlight!) they need to grow and thrive. Stunted herbs are much more susceptible to disease and pest infestation as well. To avoid this, weed your garden beds thoroughly when establishing them. If you are using a preexisting garden space that already has soil filled with weeds, keep two things in mind: (1) soil filled with weeds likely means the soil is healthy and has the nutrients present to successfully grow your herbs garden, and (2) pull the weeds as far in advance as you can (I begin weeding as soon as the soil has thawed in late winter), removing the entire root system whenever possible. Once your garden is established, make a conscious effort to take ten minutes every day or so to walk through the garden and pull out any weeds that have sprouted before they have an opportunity to invade and suffocate your herbs, or go to seed and multiply. Weeding is a satisfying and therapeutic task, and the perfect way to leave your garden at the end of each day.

Harden Off

If you have chosen to grow from seed indoors, you will want to harden off your seedlings, which means to acclimate them to the outdoor temperature, amount of light and humidity, and other environmental conditions before transplanting them outdoors. After all threat of frost has passed, gradually begin exposing them to the outdoor environment over a period of several days. I start by opening the greenhouse doors and letting the natural air temperature fill the space for a couple days. For a couple days following, I move the seedling trays and pots just outside my greenhouse and into an area with sunlight for two hours mid-day. Every couple of days after that, I extend the amount of time they are outdoors. By day ten, they are ready to move to their permanent home in the garden. Continue to nurture your seedlings as they develop strength through their leaves and root systems. Remember, take care of them now, and they will take care of *you* later.

Support

While herbs don't typically need too much support, I recommend having some wooden rods on hand because, inevitably, some herbs will grow a foot overnight and will leave you scrambling. For nasturtium, which trails, I recommend making a simple teepee by collecting three wooden rods, about three feet long each, and pushing them into the soil about twelve inches apart and twelve inches deep in a triangle formation. Using twine, bend the top ends together and tie them securely. This will allow your nasturtium to climb vertically up each leg of the teepee. I use bamboo for all my teepees, but foraged wind-blown branches work just as well, though they may not last as many seasons. A single wooden rod will suffice for herbs like fennel that may need minor vertical support. And a pocketful of small tomato clips come in super handy as well.

Planting

Strategically planting your herbs with consideration of growing conditions and tendencies as well as accessibility and physical characteristics can improve the growth, flavor, and health of the plants in your herb garden. I recommend considering which herbs prefer similar growing conditions (for example, full versus partial shade or preferred soil moisture levels) and planting those herbs together. It's also important to consider the expected height of the plant when full grown. Plant the tallest plants, like sweet marjoram, in the back so that they don't cast shade on the shorter plants and so that all the plants are easily accessible for harvesting. Herbs that vine or trail, such as nasturtium, should be planted near a trellis. Take a moment to guide their tendrils around the trellis once to start them off in the right direction. I recommend that herbs with invasive growing tendencies, such as mint, be planted in their own containers, as well as trouble-making herbs, such as eucalyptus and fennel. Herbs that require the most watering should be planted closest to the water spigot or at the base of the drip irrigation line. You may also wish to zone your plants based on their purpose and how often you use them and tend to them. For example, if you plan to snip fresh culinary herbs all summer and fall, create a zone or designate a bed close to your home or kitchen that is dedicated to kitchen herbs. Within that zone, plant your culinary herbs according to height, with the shortest herbs around the border and the tallest herbs in the center or back.

Companion Planting

Strategically planting herbs, with consideration for how they repel insects and promote or inhibit the growth of other herbs in your garden, can lead to a more diverse and healthier garden ecosystem, as well as improve the taste and yield of your harvests. Below are some of the most popular herb companion planting tips I've found useful:

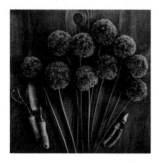

Allium This striking perennial herb, with its purple, globe-shaped, lacy head of tiny edible flowers, is valued for its culinary, ornamental, and medicinal properties but also acts as a great pest deterrent. Its pungent odor deters aphids and slugs. Plant with anything but fennel.

Basil This herb can be grown with borage, chamomile, cilantro, dill, lemon balm, nasturtium, parsley, oregano, and yarrow, but avoid planting it with fennel and sage, as they can inhibit each other's growth.

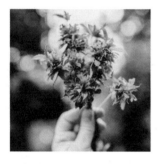

Bee balm A versatile herb that can be grown with a variety of other herbs, including catnip, calendula, lavender, oregano, rose, sage, and thyme, which all prefer well-draining soil and full sun. Avoid growing bee balm near basil, fennel (alters flavor), or parsley. Bee balm repels aphids, spider mites, Japanese beetles, and mosquitoes.

Borage Very friendly and can be planted with anything. It is an especially good companion for basil, improving its growth and flavor.

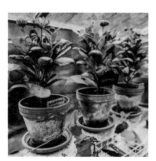

Calendula This beautiful herb grows nicely in many herb gardens next to a variety of herbs, especially bee balm, chamomile, dill, and yarrow.

Catnip An excellent repellent of ants, aphids, Japanese beetles, flea beetles, and many other insects, and can be planted with any herb except parsley, which does not grow well with any member of the mint family. It is most beneficial as a companion to chive, lavender, and rose.

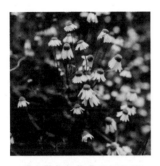

Chamomile This herb is an excellent companion to basil, lavender, and rosemary, as it helps increase the oil production of these herbs, making them more potent. It is also a good companion to calendula. Avoid planting with mint (which has invasive tendencies) or fennel (which can alter the flavor of other herbs around it).

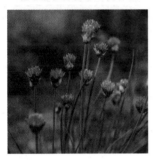

Chive Repels aphids and gets along well with pretty much every herb I can think of except fennel. I recommend growing chive with basil, cilantro, and parsley, which all prefer moist, rich soil, and tolerate partial shade.

79

Cilantro Avoid planting with fennel (alters flavor). Instead, pair with basil, chive, dill, and lavender. Repels spider mites and aphids.

Dill This herb prefers acidic soil, so it should not be planted with lavender, which prefers alkaline soil. Also do not plant near fennel, which can drastically change the flavor of dill. Basil, calendula, cilantro, lemon balm, and marigold are great companions.

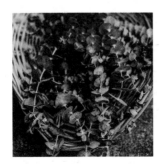

Eucalyptus Technically an evergreen but often used and referred to as an herb, eucalyptus should be planted alone, as the leaves and roots inhibit other plants from growing near them due to naturally occurring chemicals. Some gardeners suggest that lavender will grow successfully near eucalyptus, but I have not tried it. Eucalyptus repels many garden pests, including mosquitoes, ants, flies, spiders, lice, even cockroaches, and is a beautiful addition to any herb and flower garden; however, it can attract many garden pests as well, including aphids and spider mites.

Fennel Should not be planted with any other herbs or vegetables, as it has been known to change the flavor of whatever grows next to it.

Juniper Much like eucalyptus, plant juniper alone, as the leaves and roots inhibit other plants from growing around them due to naturally occurring chemicals. Some gardeners suggest that lavender can successfully grow near juniper, but I have not tried it. Juniper oil is an effective pest repellent, deterring mosquitoes, ticks, and fleas, but the plant also attracts garden pests such as aphids and spider mites, which is another reason to plant it away from herbs and vegetables.

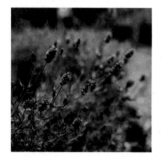

Lavender A lovely herb that prefers alkaline soil and repels moths, fleas, and mosquitoes. Plant with chamomile, marigold, oregano, rose, rosemary, sage, thyme, and yarrow. Avoid planting with mint and dill, which prefers more acidic soil.

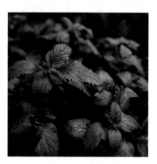

Lemon Balm Grows well near basil, dill, and nasturtium. It deters cabbage moths, mosquitoes, and gnats, so I recommend planting it by itself in a pot that can be easily moved to tabletops and near seating areas to keep mosquitoes from disrupting your garden parties.

Marigold One of the most well-known insect-repelling plants, marigold is an excellent companion plant to thyme. Together they create a barrier against garden pests. Marigold is also a good companion to cilantro, dill, lavender, rose, and rosemary.

Mint Repels ants, aphids, flea beetles, and whiteflies. While it gets along with pretty much all herbs except parsley, it is extremely invasive, so I recommend giving mint its own dedicated planter.

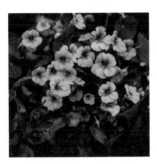

Nasturtium Best known for being a trap crop in the garden, nasturtium is often planted next to basil, lemon balm, or oregano, luring aphids, slugs, and other pests away from them.

Oregano Repels mosquitoes, so I recommend planting it in a small pot that can be easily moved to tabletops and near seating areas to keep mosquitoes from pestering your garden guests. Oregano is also a good companion for basil, lavender, thyme, and yarrow, and appreciates rubbing elbows with nasturtium too.

Parsley Repels thrips, aphids, and spongy moths. Plant with chive, cilantro, and other shade-tolerant herbs, as well as basil. Avoid growing parsley near all members of the mint family.

81

Rose This beautiful and useful shrub, often used and referred to as an herb, is susceptible to many pests in the garden, including aphids, Japanese beetles, fuller rose beetles, spider mites, thrips, rose chafers, rose slugs, rose sawflies, and leafhoppers, among others. For this reason, roses are commonly planted with herbs such as catnip, lavender, marigold, rosemary, sage, thyme, and yarrow, which repel pests with their potent scents.

Rosemary Repels many garden pests, including slugs, snails, and mosquitoes, but should only be planted with chamomile, lavender, marigold, rose, sage, and yarrow.

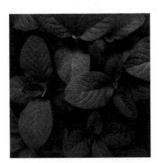

Sage Repels snails, cabbage moths, and flea beetles and is a good companion to lavender, rose, and rosemary, but should not be planted near any other herbs.

St. John's wort Repels aphids and other common garden pests. It is a good companion to cabbage and kale because it repels cabbage moth. It is an excellent addition to any garden, inviting birds, bees, and butterflies to visit throughout the summer.

Thyme Repels whiteflies and cabbage moths and is a good companion to lavender, oregano, rose, and yarrow, all dry soil lovers. Avoid planting near mint (invasive) or basil, which prefers more moist and nutrient-dense soil than thyme.

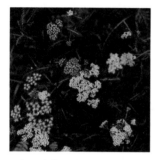

Yarrow A pest-resistant herb that attracts beneficial insects such as butterflies, ladybugs, and hoverflies, as well predatory wasps, which drink the nectar and then use garden pests as food for their larvae. Yarrow is a good companion to basil, calendula, cilantro, lavender, oregano, rose, rosemary, and thyme. Yarrow also has deep roots that reach into the subsoil for potassium, calcium, and magnesium, improving soil, which directly benefits all the other plants around it. Just be careful, as yarrow can become invasive if left unchecked. Shear them to the ground to contain them.

Container-Grown Herbs

Growing herbs in containers is a wonderful way to add fresh flavors and fragrances to indoor and outdoor gathering spaces and allows for a wider variety of herbs to be grown in small spaces. It is a great solution in limited-space situations, when tending a garden is not possible, or if the ground in your space is contaminated. Containers also offer the advantage of portability, providing the flexibility to relocate your herbs in the event of harsh weather. Nearly any herb can be grown in a container or window box. Culinary herbs such as basil, thyme, mint, rosemary, and parsley are just a few of the many varieties that thrive in pots, making it easy to create your own personal herb garden while reining in herbs with invasive tendencies. Herbs that repel mosquitoes are particularly ideal for containers, so they can easily be placed near seating areas and gathering spaces. Another benefit of container gardening is that, if you want to grow an herb that requires very different soil than what is in your growing beds, you have a much smaller volume of soil to amend. Containers are also a great way to add personal style to your garden, elements of natural, living design, and pops of color and texture to other outdoor living areas like porches, terraces, balconies, and gazebos. Time-worn pieces, such as glazed ceramics and terracotta, are traditional and timeless container types that provide striking contrast to the rich green colors of most herbs and come in wide varieties of colors, textures, and sizes. And repurposing your favorite vintage finds, like old, galvanized bins and buckets, half-barrels, metal milk cans, old milk crates, baskets, tea pots, butter crocks, metal toolboxes, and metal chicken feeders and waterers, is another way to add character and a level of interest to your garden or outdoor living space, and the results often become conversation pieces for your guests.

Keep in mind that the type of material the container is made of can alter the amount of water it holds. For example, terracotta naturally wicks water away, making it an ideal material for those, like me, in regions that receive a lot of precipitation, but do require you to water more frequently during dry spells and are more likely to crack. Glazed ceramics, on the other hand, naturally retain moisture and are less likely to crack during the winter. Galvanized metal containers are sturdy options that can be found in several shapes and sizes, but typically don't have good drainage. The good news is, drill a handful of holes with the electric screwdriver and problem solved!

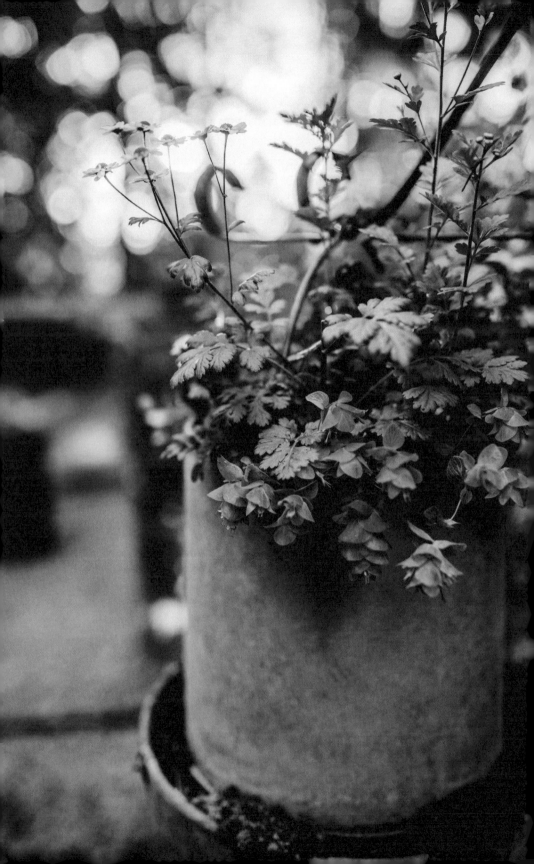

Tips for Container Planting with Herbs

- If you plan to use a nontraditional pot that doesn't already have holes in the bottom, be sure that there are enough rusted-through holes or cracks to provide adequate drainage, or drill holes if needed.

- Take into consideration how much the herb will spread when choosing its container. Some herbs, like mint, yarrow, and St. John's wort, have underground root systems that spread quickly and will need lots of growing space, while other herbs like parsley, basil, rosemary, and chive do not need as much.

- Add a layer of pebbles to the bottom for additional drainage.

- Use a saucer under pots to help retain water during the hottest months, but remove it during the wet seasons.

- Use a good fluffy potting mix to fill containers, *not* garden soil.

- Check the moisture level of the soil daily during the hottest and driest months of the year.

- Always replenish the soil at the beginning of each new growing season, adding to the top of each bed or container as needed, and working it into the top few inches of existing soil.

- Feed your containers with an organic fertilizer every two weeks.

- Move containers out of direct sun on the hottest summer days.

- Move containers to a cooler space with partial shade if you are going away for the weekend.

- Use platforms on casters (wheels) to assist in moving heavy containers.

With the right soil, water, fertilizer, and light conditions, container herbs can flourish and provide an abundant supply of delicious herbs for cooking, botanical cocktails, self-care products, and aromatherapy, and can easily be brought inside when the season turns.

Protect from Pests

Once your starts have moved to their permanent home, keep a close eye out for garden pests, and take steps to control them using organic methods when they are first identified. Aphids and slugs do the most damage in my garden, and I've found that home remedies such as diluted dish-soap solutions go a long way to keeping these pests under control. Small mesh bags of ladybugs (usually several hundred to a single bag) can sometimes be purchased at your local garden center and released into areas with aphid activity. Ladybugs are extremely efficient at halting aphid infestation. In fact, a single ladybug can eat up to sixty aphids a day! It is recommended you have, at the very minimum, two ladybugs for every square foot of garden space.

Nutrients

While herbs don't usually require a lot of fertilizer, it is a good idea to give them a boost of supplemental nutrition on a regular basis. Even though I have good soil with a high organic content, I still fertilize established plants every two weeks, using a general-purpose fertilizer or fish emulsion, to ensure that I continue to grow high-yielding plants and that my harvests are high in nutritional value. Just make sure it's organic, since you'll ingest these herbs and/or use them on your skin.

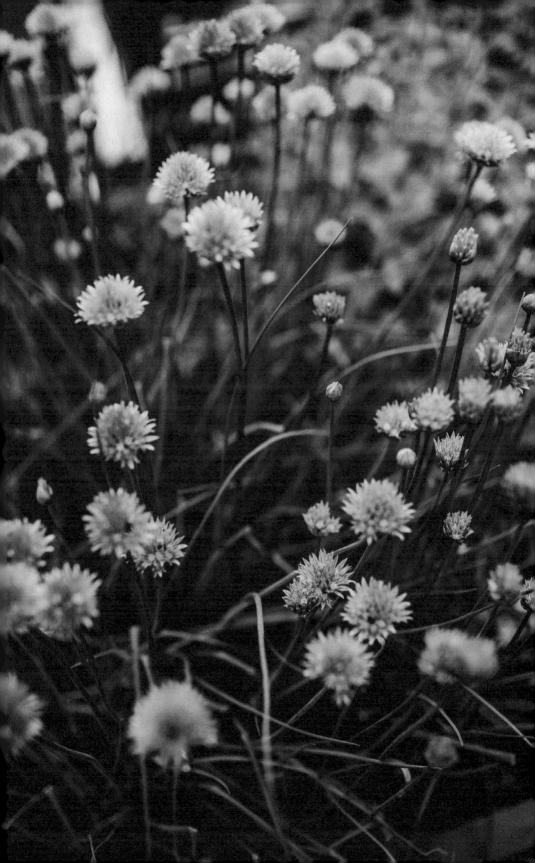

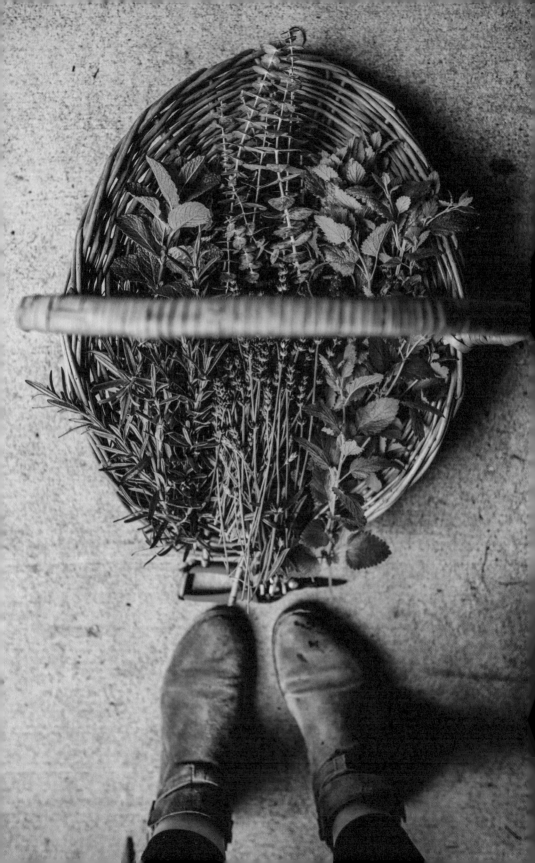

Part II

Gather + Keep

"How delightful it is to walk in a garden,
and to gather the herbs and flowers
which the bountiful hand of Nature
has scattered with such lavish profusion."

*—Charlotte Campbell Bury,
The Lady's Own Cookery Book (1775–1861)*

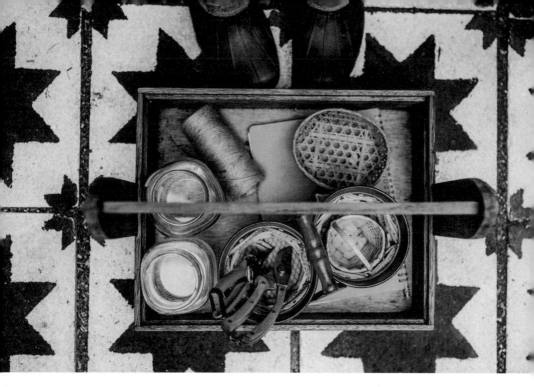

Harvesting

Harvesting herbs is an important step in maintaining a healthy and productive garden. These tips can help ensure that your herb garden remains healthy and productive throughout the growing season, while you enjoy bountiful harvests.

A Harvester's Toolkit

- Clean, sharp snips and/or pruning shears

- Baskets in various sizes for collecting blossom heads, such as calendula, marigold, and chamomile

- Jars of clean, cold water to hold stems that you want to keep fresh

- Twine to tie stems for drying

- Utility cart or wagon for bountiful harvests

- Garden journal and pencil to document harvests and other observations from your garden visit

- Camera so you can document the beautiful herbs and garden space you have cultivated

Time of Day

The time of day at which you harvest your herbs can greatly impact the amount of essential oils and medicinal properties in the plant. The best time to harvest herbs is in the morning, after the dew has evaporated, but before the sun has hit the aerial parts of the plant for too long. This is when the largest percentage of beneficial properties (flavor and fragrance and oils, for example) are in the plant. As the heat from the sun sets in, those properties slowly drain back into the stem and roots of the plant. If you are foraging, be mindful not to harvest endangered or at-risk plants, and never take more than you need at one time. Robin Wall Kimmerer said it best in *Braiding Sweetgrass*: "The honorable harvest. Take only what you need and use everything you take."

Use Sharp Snips

Use sharp, clean snips or pruning shears to harvest your herbs, as dull blades can damage the plant and make it more susceptible to disease. My husband purchased a twelve-dollar utility sharpener online, and it does a great job sharpening my snips every month or so. I clean them often with a spray bottle of rubbing alcohol that I keep in the greenhouse. For snips, I recommend a pair with red handles so you can easily find them when you leave them in a garden bed. Trust me on this.

Cut Above a Leaf Node

When harvesting, cut the stem above a leaf node or pair of leaves. This will encourage the plant to produce new growth and prevent it from becoming too woody.

Don't Remove More Than a Third of the Plant

To ensure the health of your herbs, avoid removing more than a third of the plant at once. This will allow the plant to continue growing and producing throughout the season.

Rinse Before Using

Once you've harvested your herbs, rinse them gently in cool water and pat dry with a paper towel before using. Keep in mind that handling and washing herbs can release and wash away the beneficial properties, such as the aroma and flavor of the herb, so handle as minimally as possible.

Keep a Journal

This is a good time to consider keeping a garden journal, where you can detail what you grew, seed sowing dates, harvesting dates with itemized lists of what was gathered, and which herbs you used and enjoyed most. Record what happens each season, as well as what garden maintenance was necessary, and include dates to make planning easier the following year. I always record the date we actually experienced our last frost of the year in addition to my zone's estimated final frost date, as the final frost date assigned to your zone

is merely a historical estimate. Also, don't be afraid to jot down your garden failures as well as your successes. What you fell in love with and want to grow more of, as well as what doesn't make the cut for next year or simply doesn't grow well in your microclimate or a particular growing space. Sketch each bed garden bed or container, labeling it with a number or name, and make a chart indicating what grew where, for plant rotation purposes or simply so you know where your perennials will pop up next spring. Don't forget to include specific variety names! (Trust me on this; I always think I will remember where all my perennials are and what varieties they are, but I never do.) Garden journaling is a calming, therapeutic process that I truly enjoy and highly recommend. During the shortest days of the year, you will find comfort in opening your journal and looking back at the past year as you begin garden dreaming for the growing season ahead.

Propagating

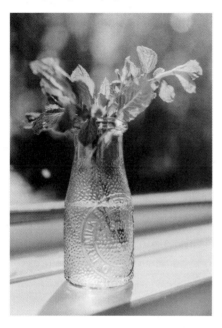

Herb gardening can get expensive, but with a cutting from your favorite herb and a glass jar of water, you can turn a single plant into a hefty supply of new ones. Propagating herbs in water is a simple method of reproducing a plant from a cutting. To propagate an herb, start by using a clean pair of shears to snip a six-to-eight-inch stem below a leaf node from a healthy, mature herb plant during the peak of its growing season (typically summer). (Remember, the best time to harvest herbs is in the morning, after the dew has evaporated but before the plant has been sun-kissed for too long, draining the nutrients it needs to generate a new root system.) Remove all leaves from the bottom two inches of the plant, and snip off any blossoms or buds so that the plant can focus all its energy on creating a new root system. Drop the stem into clean water in a glass jar, ensuring that there are no leaves submerged in water. Keep the jar in a warm place (68–72 degrees Fahrenheit) and make sure it has some indirect sunlight throughout the day. Over time, the stem should grow new roots, becoming a new plant all its own. Keep in mind that not every stem will propagate, so take a few cuttings from every plant that you wish to root. If your jar is large enough, you can combine a few stems of the same plant in a single jar.

I enjoy setting up a mini propagation station of water jars on my kitchen windowsill so I can watch the roots take form over time and keep the water fresh, changing it out every two to four days as needed to prevent algae and bacteria from forming. Depending on the type of plant you are propagating and the conditions you're propagating in, rooting can take anywhere from a few days to several months, but two to four weeks is typical for most herbs. Once the herb has an established root system (several roots that are two inches long or more), you can continue to grow it in the water and begin harvesting the leaves for culinary and medicinal uses, sizing up the jars as needed to hold the growing root base. Alternatively, if you'd like to transplant the herb plant into an outdoor garden bed, first transplant it into a pot of soil on the windowsill to give it time to adjust to living in soil before transplanting it outdoors. While propagating herbs is not as convenient as buying starter plants at the nursery that already have an established root system in soil, it is much less expensive and is a great way to continue growing during the colder months. It is, however, faster than growing the same herb from seed. It is also a convenient way to keep living culinary herbs readily available in your kitchen without the mess of potting soil and pests, such as fungus gnats, which are drawn to moist soil conditions.

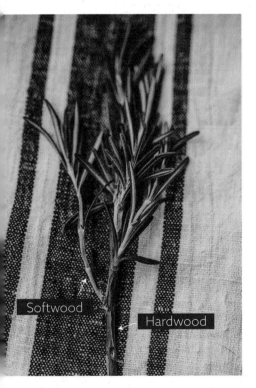

Softwood

Hardwood

Rooting in water works especially well for soft-stemmed herbs such as mint, basil, lemon balm, parsley, and lemon grass. You can successfully propagate woody-stemmed herbs like rosemary, oregano, thyme, and sage in water as well, but you will want to take the cuttings from the new green growth of the plant, known as the "softwood" section, not the older woody stem of the plant, known as the "hardwood" section, and be prepared for them to take a month or more to root. As a side note, I have not had luck propagating cilantro or dill in water, and recommend starting those from seed.

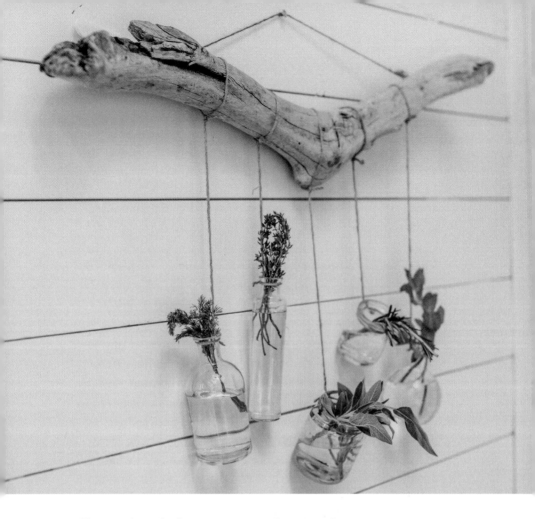

Driftwood and Glass Propagation Station

If you don't have windowsill space to spare, consider creating a simple hanging station. It is a beautiful way to add life and color to a bare wall during the propagation process.

You Will Need

piece of driftwood (or branch of your choosing)

jute twine

small glass jars with lips (one for each stem you wish to propagate)

2 picture hangers (optional)

fresh herb stems

To Make

1. Cut a piece of twine thirty-six inches long and tie the ends around each end of the driftwood, double-knot to secure it, and snip the excess twine ends. This is your hanger. Alternatively, you can screw picture hangers into the back of your driftwood, approximately two inches in from each end, and then double-knot your twine to them to create the hanger.

2. Cut one piece of eighteen-inch twine for each jar you want to incorporate. Tie one end of the eighteen-inch twine around the top of the glass jar so that the twine sits snugly under the lip. Double-knot the twine tightly. Repeat this step for every jar.

3. Secure each jar to the driftwood, letting them hang below. Space them evenly between the end ties from step one, and stagger the heights of the jars so they don't bump each other when hanging. Snip off excess jute from the ends for a clean look.

4. Now your station is ready to hang! Loop the twine hanger once around a nail or hook in the wall to prevent it from shifting or sliding. You can also add a command strip to the back of the driftwood for added support. The driftwood should lie flat against the wall. Alternatively, it could hang on a hook or nail above a window, so it hangs over the window pane.

5. Once your station is hung, use a narrow-spouted watering can to fill the bottles three-quarters full with clean cool water.

6. Condition your herb stems by cutting them in the softwood area and removing the bottom half of the leaves. Drop the stems into the water, ensuring that no leaves are submerged.

Note: Algae will grow faster in clear glass jars than in colored or opaque glass jars; however, I still prefer to use clear glass jars, so I can see the roots forming and monitor the water. As long as you change out the water frequently, algae won't have a chance to grow. If algae begins to grow despite these efforts, untie the jar, empty and clean it thoroughly, and retie it back onto the driftwood before refilling it with fresh water and dropping your herb stem(s) back in.

Preserving

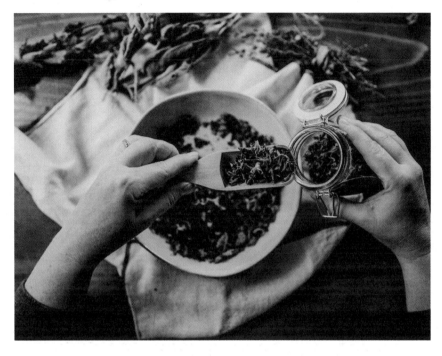

"Time is an herb that cures all diseases."

—*Benjamin Franklin* (1705–1790)

Regardless of how you choose to preserve your herbs, first wash them gently in cool water to remove any soil or insects. With a clean pair of shears (or your fingers) snip or tear off any leaves or parts of the plant that are blemished or have been nibbled. Then shake the plants to remove the majority of the water. Pat dry with a paper towel and let dry completely, so no moisture is visible. Preserving herbs can be a peaceful, slow, fragrant task.

If you have more herbs than you can use fresh, consider these methods for preserving them so they can be enjoyed year-round. Herbs that are dried or frozen can keep up to a year; however, they may begin to lose their potency after six months.

Drying

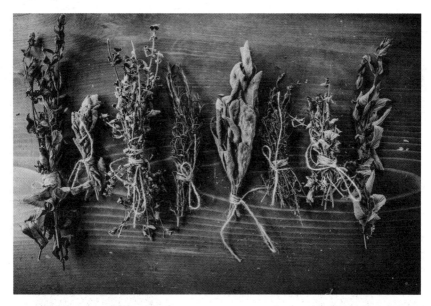

Lay your herbs in a single layer on a mesh drying rack to dry, or bundle a few sprigs together with jute twine (tied tightly) and hang. I usually do a combination of both. Dry in a warm, dry, airy location with good circulation. I keep a dehumidifier running near the drying rack to help remove moisture from the air near where the herbs are drying and to keep the air continuously circulating. Alternatively, you can use a dehydrator to dry your herbs in a more expedited manner.

Make sure your herbs are completely dry before storing them in clean, airtight jars. If air-drying, I typically check them at about the two-week mark and go from there. They should have a brittle texture and crumble easily. Some will be ready to jar, while others will need more time. Spreading them out so they aren't touching speeds up the drying process a bit.

Strip leaves and flowers from the main stem and store them in their whole form, when possible, to preserve potency. Beneficial properties are released when they are broken or crushed, so crush with a mortar and pestle (or with your hands) right before using them.

Label your jars with the variety of herb you're storing and the date of harvest. Most herbs will maintain their flavor and potency for twelve to eighteen months. If you notice that your herbs lack luster (no longer smell potent or the color is fading), use them to make botanical fire starters (page 287) or simply compost them back into the earth. Store the jars in a cool, dry area away from direct sunlight.

My Favorite Herbs to Dry

- Basil
- Bay
- Bee balm
- Butterfly pea
- Calendula
- Chamomile
- Echinacea

- Eucalyptus
- Feverfew
- Lavender
- Lemon balm
- Marigold
- Mint
- Oregano

- Rose
- Rosemary
- Sage
- Thyme
- Yarrow

Freezing

Freezing is often considered the best way to preserve herbs that have delicate flavors or textures, or that have tender leaves. Dill, chive, cilantro, and parsley are examples of herbs that preserve best when frozen, but all herbs can be preserved using this process. My favorite herb-freezing method uses an ice cube tray. Chop the herbs into small pieces and evenly distribute across the tray. Then pour water or organic extra virgin olive oil over the herbs. Carefully relocate to the freezer. Once the oil cubes are frozen, pop them out and store in a plastic bag in the freezer for up to a year to be used individually as needed. Herb and water cubes can be thawed and drained. Herb and oil cubes can be dropped straight onto your skillet. This freezing method can also be used to portion out and preserve homemade pesto!

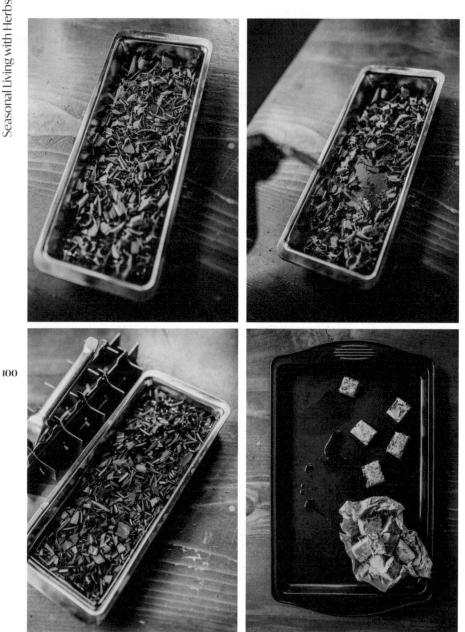

Pictured: a versatile herb blend of rosemary, sage, and thyme in extra virgin olive oil

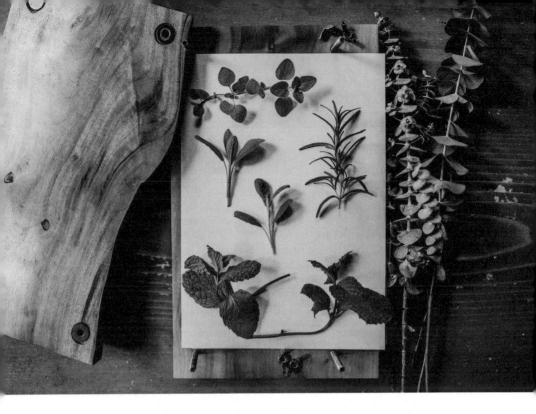

Pressing

While I understand that the process of pressing flowers can be expedited in a microwave or oven, I prefer the more traditional method of pressure and time. A few times a week, during the spring and summer months, I find myself harvesting specifically to press and preserve, most of the time without a specific purpose in mind. Pressed flowers take up nearly no space, will keep for decades, and are quite literally a method of preserving a botanical moment in time. Here are some of my favorite, tried-and-true botanical pressing tips.

Before harvesting, be sure you have allotted yourself enough time to press as well. Some plants will begin to wilt or brown shortly after harvesting, so you want to press the same day, preferably the same hour. Avoid harvesting herbs when they are wet with dew or rain, or right after watering. Late morning is ideal. Search for blooms that are unblemished, meaning they have not started to brown or shrivel on the edges and are free of tears and bug nibbles. I also recommend harvesting at different stages in the plant's growing process for variety and visual interest.

What You'll Need

fresh herbs (blooms and foliage)
pair of snips for trimming
couch sheets[8]

blotting paper
tweezers
botanical press[9]

How to Press

1. Source your botanicals. Dab flowers and stems dry before pressing to remove any extra moisture. Snip off any leaves or petals you don't want to include in the press.

2. Prep your press by stacking a bottom board (corrugated cardboard works great here), followed by a piece of couch paper and then a piece of blotting paper.

3. Place herbs face down as you stack, adjusting the petals and leaves as needed. It will help the petals to press into place in a more natural way. Curve your stems and leaves into interesting positions.

4. Cover your herbs with another piece of blotting paper, then another piece of couch paper.

5. Repeat this layering system for as many herbs as you have to press.

6. Carefully place your press cover on and secure it.

7. Pressing flowers takes time. Check in on your pressed botanicals every two weeks and decide what can be removed and what should stay another week. Use tweezers to carefully transfer pressed flowers from the press to your storage box.

Note: Extremely dense-centered flowers, such as roses, will need dismantling. This is the process of deconstructing the flower and pressing the petals separately, with the intention of reassembling the pressed petals afterward to reconstruct the bloom.

8   Couch sheets are made of soft, thick paper that is designed and treated to absorb water. They are placed between the layers of botanicals and are reusable. Blotting paper is placed between the couch sheets on both sides of the botanicals to absorb excess moisture and act as a barrier between the plants and the couch sheets. This ultra-thin tissue-like paper also makes it easier to remove the herbs without damaging petals or structure.

9   If you do not have a flower press, a heavy book will do. Alternatively, you can make a quick flower press with two flat pieces of wood and a large Velcro strap, stretchy fabric, clamps, or any mechanism that will tightly secure the layers of pages and botanicals between the two boards. Better yet, you can make your own using the tutorial in the following section!

My Favorite Herbs for Pressing

- Bee balm
- Borage
- Butterfly pea
- Calendula
- Chamomile
- Dill
- Eucalyptus (silver dollar)
- Fennel
- Feverfew
- Lavender
- Lemon balm
- Marigold (French)
- Mint
- Nasturtium
- Pansy
- Rose (dismantled)
- Sage
- Viola
- Violet
- Yarrow

Store your pressed botanicals in a dry, cool, and dark place to preserve their color and shape, and in an airtight container to prevent them from being exposed to air and moisture. Avoid exposing your pressed botanicals to direct sunlight or high humidity, which can cause them to fade and discolor over time.

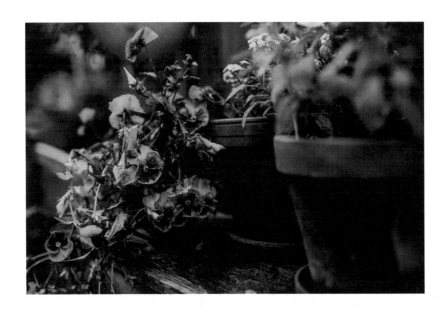

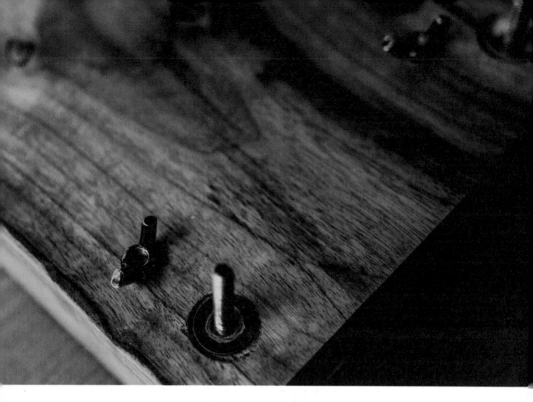

Making a Botanical Press

> "How could such sweet and wholesome hours be reckoned but in herbs and flowers?"
>
> —*Andrew Marvell*, English poet (1621–1678)

One of the most beautiful Mother's Day gifts I've ever received was a botanical press handmade by my husband. Made of live edge, air-dried walnut and finished with a French polish and wax, it literally took my breath away! Until then, I had used whatever heavy books I could find around the house to press botanicals. More often than not, I forgot about them, only to stumble upon the pressed garden gifts years later (which is always a pleasant surprise!). As a little girl, I remember pressing flowers in my family's Encyclopedia Britannica set.

/Part II: Gather + Keep

You Will Need

2 one-inch-thick flat wood pieces
4 four-inch-long carriage bolts
8 washers to fit the carriage bolts

4 wing nuts to fit the
  carriage bolts

To Make

1. Cut two pieces of wood to the same size. Though not necessary, I recommend sanding all sides and edges of each piece of wood if they're rough, so they don't cause splinters.

2. Using a permanent marker, mark a dot 1½ inches in and down from the outside edge of each corner of each piece of wood. When the pieces are stacked on top of each other, the four dots on the outside of one piece of wood should align with the four dots on the outside of the second piece of wood.

3. Using a Forstner bit that is the diameter of your washers, drill a 1/8-inch recess directly over each of the four dots on each outside piece of wood. (This step is optional, but is helpful because it centers your washers, giving them a recessed pocket to rest in.)

4. Next, drill a hole through the center of each recessed pocket that is of slightly larger diameter than your carriage bolt. For example, for a ¼-inch diameter screw, drill using a 3/8-inch diameter drill bit. When you're done, you should have four holes in each piece of wood that align when stacked.

5. Slide a washer onto each of your four bolts and, beginning underneath the bottom piece of wood, thread the bolts up through each of the four drilled holes. Then align the holes of the second piece of wood, threading the bolts up through the second set of four holes, so the pieces of wood stack like a sandwich.

6. Thread the last four washers on the top of the press. They should sit perfectly inside the recessed pocket. Then thread the wing nuts through to complete the press functionality.

7. Once everything fits and you have confirmed that the holes align, remove the hardware temporarily to finish the wood with a finish of your choice for durability and protection. (My husband used a natural oil and beeswax blend.)

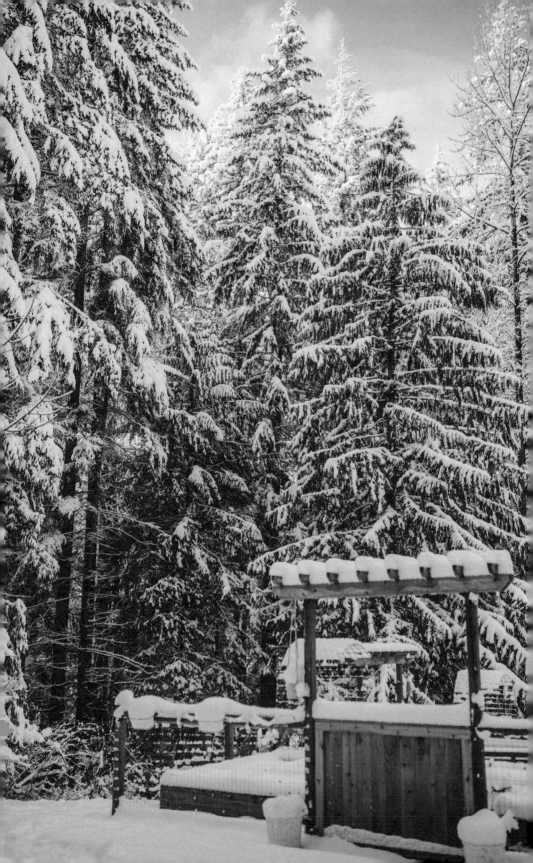

Winterizing

"This garden wasn't sleeping. It was very much awake."

—*Kate Morton, The Forgotten Garden*

For me, autumn is a time to prepare the garden for a restful winter sleep. Unlike many, I find great joy in this part of gardening. It is therapeutic to collect seeds, clear and tidy my garden beds, and tuck my perennials in for their winter nap. It gives me an opportunity to truly appreciate the cyclical journey I take with my garden, from germinating seeds to nurturing seedlings to cultivating flowers and herbs to harvesting them, and then collecting their seeds to begin the process once again. Winterizing my garden is a nod to the life cycle of each and every plant I grew that year.

Below is a list of garden tasks to tackle before winter settles in.

107

Collect Seeds

This simple act truly is a promise of next year's garden. It costs nothing but your time and is the final step in the lifestyle of your garden herbs. Calendula, bee balm, poppy, and nasturtium are great seeds for the beginner collector.

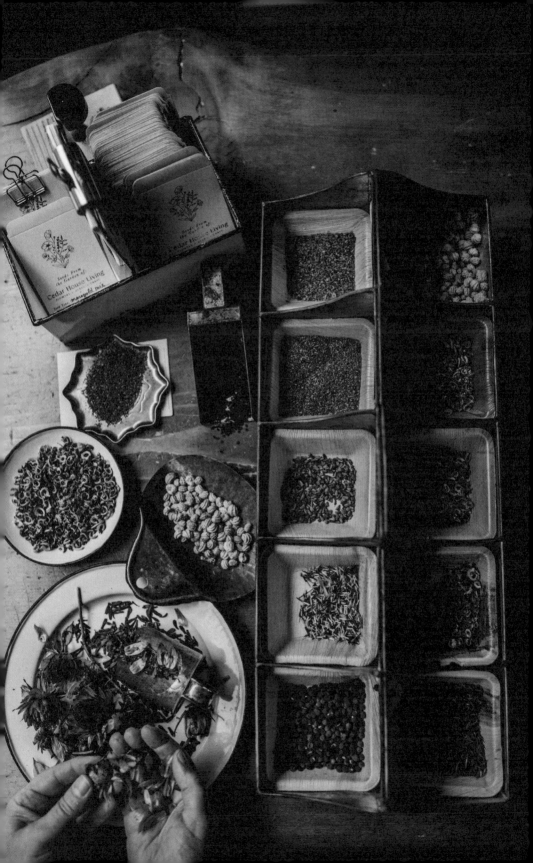

Seed Organization

There are endless ways to organize your seeds, but I will share the process and storage that works best for me.

Number of Sowings Divide your seed packs into two categories: seeds you plan to succession-sow year-round (for example, if you plan to grow basil or cilantro throughout the year indoors) and seeds you will only sow once a year in the spring for outdoor planting. The year-round seeds can be alphabetized and set aside in a rubber-banded stack. (If you don't plan to grow any herbs year-round, then skip this step entirely.)

Direct versus Indirect Sowing Using the seeds you plan to grow just once a year in the spring, divide them into one pile for seeds you plan to direct-sow, and another pile for seeds you plan to start early indoors and plant out after the last frost. The direct-sow seed packs can be alphabetized and set aside in a rubber-banded stack.

Sow Date Next, with the seeds you plan to start indoors, determine the number of weeks out you need to sow, from the back of your seed packet or your seed supplier's website, and count backward from your zone's last frost date. Do this for all the seeds in this pile, and group them by their general start-date timeframe. Keep in mind that herbs of the same genus may have very different sow dates across species and variety, so each type of seed should be calculated individually. Write that date on a sticky note and rubber-band each stack. As an example, my last frost date is April 20. If the back of my seed packet indicates that I should sow the seeds four to five weeks before my last frost date, then the approximate sow date for that seed is March 20.

Storage Now you are ready to store your organized piles of seed packs. Procure some kind of seed organization container. For a small collection of seed packets, a pretty vintage recipe box would be ideal and can be found at most flea markets or thrift stores. You can make or purchase recipe box dividers to label the seed packs by category and date, as indicated in steps one through three above. For more extensive collections of seed packs, I recommend a photo storage case. They come with several small containers that are perfectly sized to hold your seeds in their separate piles. These can be purchased online or found at your local craft store. Vintage cassette tape holders would also make really cool seed packet organizers if you happen to see one at an antique store.

Labeling I use masking tape to label each container with the sow date of each set of seed packs inside, or with "Year-Round Sow" or "Direct Sow." Place the year-round and direct-sow containers in the first slots of the case, followed by the dated organizers. If you have several varieties of the same type of herb, for example calendula, that have the same seed-starting date, you can dedicate an organizer just to them, labeling accordingly, and putting in the slot following the date. Your early-spring self will thank you for taking the time to do this in the winter when you are packaging your fall seeds or purchasing new ones.

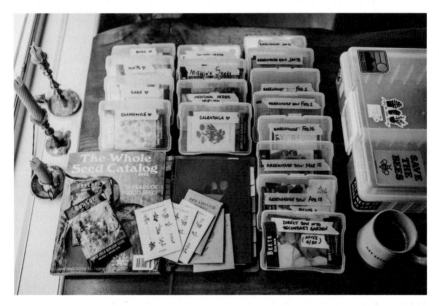

Clean Up

Clean the garden beds by removing all spent material. Pull and compost annual herbs such as basil, borage, calendula, chamomile, marigold, and nasturtium, and identify diseased plants to remove and burn or trash, including any diseased perennials.

Cut Back

Some perennials should be cut back in autumn to prevent disease and pest problems from lingering into your new season. Sharpen your shears, spray them with rubbing alcohol, and cut the plants back to about two to three inches above ground level. Here is a list of the perennials in my garden that I cut back to their basal foliage (two to three inches above the base of the plant): anise hyssop, bee balm, mint, lemon balm, lavender, chive, feverfew, oregano, lemongrass, mint, sweet marjoram (six inches above ground), yarrow, and echinacea.

Prune

Some perennials should be pruned, but not cut all the way back to the ground. Here is a list of the perennials I prune, being cautious not to remove more than a third of the plant): lavender, rose, oregano, and thyme.

Leave Standing

Some perennials should be left standing. Here is a list of perennials I do not cut back or prune during the fall/winter: rosemary, St. John's wort, sage, and eucalyptus.

Rose Care

Roses need special care at this time. There are the four primary things to remember when winterizing your rose bushes: (1) remove any foliage still hanging on from the fall, (2) completely remove any stems that show signs of damage, disease, or rot, (3) cut the shrub back to two-thirds of its size (removing the outer and uppermost third of the plant), and (4) always prune on an angle so the "top" of the clipped angle is on the outside of the plant. This will allow the plant to grow in a more visually pleasing rounded shape.

> "You must prune to bloom. If the dead weight is not pruned and removed, it compromises the quality, performance, and output of the vine. When you prune what's not working in your life, you make the space and place for renewal to happen and for new growth to spring forth."
>
> —*Susan C. Young*, American author

Transplant

Autumn is the time for transplanting perennials that you wish to overwinter into large containers and relocating them to their winter abode. For me, it's a greenhouse, but for others, it may be a porch, balcony, garage, or even a window in your home with good sun exposure.

Plant New

If you are adding new shrubs or perennials to your garden or landscape, plant these in the autumn to give them an ample dormant period before their first spring bloom in their new home.

Tuck Them In

Now that your beds are tidied and your herbs are trimmed, it's time to tuck them in for the winter. Begin by removing all support pieces, which should be soaked in, or sprayed with, a one-to-two ratio solution of bleach to water before storing them away. This will kill any diseases lingering on the supports, so they don't follow you into the new growing year.

Next, spread a heavy layer of compost over the garden beds, except for the areas immediately surrounding any new shrubs or perennials you have just planted. Composted manure, packed with nutrients that your garden needs, is truly the perfect winter blanket. Fall is the best time to add composted manure to your garden, allowing plenty of time for the manure to properly break down so that it doesn't burn your starts next spring.

Finally, collect fallen leaves from your property, crumble them (or rake them into a pile and run them over a few times with the lawn mower to quickly chop them), and mix them into your top layer of compost. This technique of incorporating leaf debris not only fills your garden with *free* organic mulch, but it will actually *nourish* your garden next year. You see, as the leaves decompose over the next year, this green material actually improves your soil, acting as a natural fertilizer. Additionally, leaves will retain moisture in your soil (less irrigation needed) *and* help suppress weeds (your back will thank you!). Lastly, leaves naturally buffer the temperature of your soil, keeping it warmer in the winter months, protecting your perennials, and cooler in the summer months, protecting your spring seedlings. A win-win situation all around.

"If you've never experienced the joy of accomplishing more than you can imagine, plant a garden."

—*Robert Brault*, American writer

113

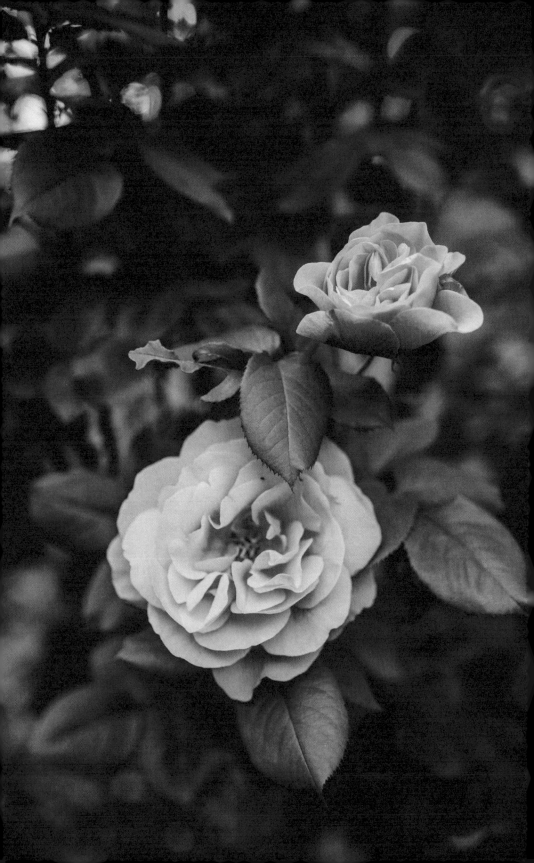

Part III

Botanically Speaking

"As a mother you'd do well to add some herb lore to your store of knowledge for you never can be sure when your children's well-being might depend upon it."

—*Geraldine Brooks, Year of Wonders*

This section of the book was developed by walking around my backyard garden and investigating, researching, and then writing about the physical attributes and growth habits of many of the herbs I grow. I do not claim to be an expert on medicinal herbs, and you do not need to be an herbalist or medical professional to appreciate, learn from, and utilize the pages that follow. Please view the following section for what it is: a collection of my research on herbal history, alongside herbal academic research, and my understanding of how these herbs have been used, how they could be used, and what beneficial properties they are said to naturally have. At the back of the book, I've included a list of all the works I consulted to create this compilation. If there is an herb that particularly interests you, I invite you to further research it on your own with specific regard to how you wish to use it.

Also included in this section are my own personal experiences, insights, and tips for growing my favorite herbs, common ways they are used, and my own favorite ways to use them. When appropriate, I've even included my personal favorite varieties of a particular herb to grow. However, I strongly advise you to consult your health care professional before consuming or topically applying any herbs that you are not familiar with.

And, last but not least, let this section be a reminder to never underestimate the usefulness, beauty, and healing power of an herb garden.

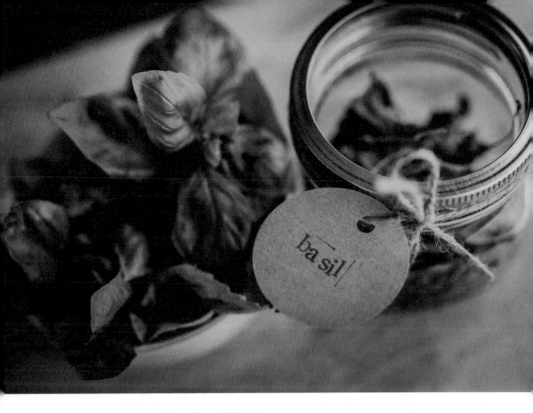

Basil *Ocimum basilicum*

"A man taking basil from a woman will love her always."

—*Thomas More*, social philosopher (1478–1535)

Belonging to the Lamiaceae (mint) family, basil (prounounced "bay-zil" or "baz-il") is an annual with fragrant leafy stems and small white late-summer flowers. The leaves are most commonly oval and green. Basil plants typically grow one to two feet tall with a bushy appearance and thrive in bright sunny areas. It is sometimes referred to as common basil, sweet basil, sweet bazil, the devil's plant, witches herb, or St. Joseph's Wort.

Beneficial Properties and Common Uses

Basil has many beneficial attributes including anti-inflammatory, antioxidant, anti-fungal, and anti-nausea properties, and is an excellent source of vitamins A, C and K, as well as calcium, magnesium, iron, phosphorus, and potassium. Basil is commonly used to support the digestive system, sooth overworked muscles (when used topically as an infused oil,) and naturally support those with upper respiratory infections, asthma, colds and flus when ingested as an herbal tea or used in a neti pot. Basil essential oil is used in aromatherapy to sooth and relax the mind after a stressful day.

Basil is most commonly grown as a kitchen herb and used in culinary preparations, with Italian tomato sauce and pesto and Thai cuisine making it most famous. Sprigs of basil, which can include their flowering buds, make beautiful and aromatic garnishes to dishes, charcuterie boards, and cocktails.

In the garden, the aroma of basil naturally repels pests, particularly mosquitos. Basil also attracts pollinators such as bees and butterflies, and is an excellent garden companion to tomatoes, even enhancing their flavor. It grows well alongside asparagus, beans, beets, eggplant, lettuces, and potatoes.

> **Precautionary Note:** Avoid using basil essential oils on children, or if pregnant or nursing, as it contains estragole CT, which is strong and can risk the safety of baby and mother.

Try basil in the recipes and tutorials on pages 196, 198, 221, 270

To Grow

Basil is a popular herb to grow in the garden, and for good reason! It is prized for its flavorful leaves and versatility and thrives in both garden beds as well as pots. It can grow outdoors or inside on a south-facing windowsill. It grows easily from seed but is quite sensitive to cold and will not withstand frost. If temperatures dip below 50 degrees, it is likely your basil plant's leaves will turn black. Direct sow basil seeds after all chance of frost have passed and soil has warmed. Choose a sunny location that receives at least six hours of direct sunlight daily, and preferably an area that has shelter from strong winds, with rich, well-draining soil. Basil is hardy in USDA zones 3-10.

If growing from seed, start indoors six to eight weeks before the last frost. Germination typically occurs in five to seven days in ideal conditions. Use a humidity dome or cover trays with plastic wrap to aid in germination. Once the seedlings emerge and grow at least one set of true leaves, thin to one seedling per cell. Pot up as needed. Transplant outside once the soil has warmed. Pinch off the top set of true leaves once the seedlings have six sets of true leaves to promote strong and busy plants.

Alternatively, starter plants are often available at your local garden center and planted out two weeks after the last frost. Basil is a great companion to tomatoes and peppers, enhancing their growth.

Finally, basil is incredibly easy to grow from cuttings. To learn more about the propagation method, visit page 93.

My Favorite Varieties

I most enjoy growing basil for its culinary uses as well as its lovely fragrant foliage additions to flower arrangements. While there are over 40 varieties of basil, below is a list of the ones I grow:

- **Genovese basil** – classic Italian variety with extra-large dark green leaves; great for culinary use

- **Sweet basil** – most common variety for culinary use; strong flavor and aroma; bold green more rounded leaves; repels mosquitos

- **Purple basil** – also known as chocolate basil or dark opal basil; dark burgundy color with pointed leaves (though my favorite are the genetic marvels that grow unique speckled or striated variations) and pink flowers; lovely clove flavor; gorgeous addition to floral arrangements

- **Italian broad leaf basil** – tall, fast-growing annual with gorgeous leaves perfect for garnishing Italian dishes and herbal cocktails

- **Cinnamon basil** – spicy, fragrant variety with hint of cinnamon flavor; stems are a reddish-purple color; flowers pink; beautiful and fragrant addition to floral arrangements

- **Thai sweet basil** – smaller pointed dark green leaves with dark purple flower head; spicy licorice flavor and aroma commonly found in Asian dishes; retains its flavor at higher cooking temperatures compared to other types of basil; beautiful and fragrant addition to floral arrangements

- **Mammoth basil** – mild-flavored extra-large ruffled lettuce-like leaves are 6-10 inches long and 4 inches wide making them perfect for using as lettuce wraps; sometimes called lettuce basil

- **Holy basil** – also called tulsi or sacred basil; highly fragrant with a spicy, sweet aroma commonly used in herbal teas; flavor is best when cooked (can be slightly bitter if eaten raw); a medicinal herb with stress-reducing benefits and used to treat stomach ailments and promote blood circulation; commonly used in mouthwashes.

Care and Harvest

Basil prefers consistently moist soil, so water regularly and mulch around the base of the plant to help retain moisture. Pinching back the tips of the plant regularly through harvesting will encourage more growth, a bushier stature, and prevent the basil from going to seed too quickly. Harvest in the morning after the dew has dried but before the sun is directly overhead to retain the greatest amount of its beneficial properties and essential oils. In the event of an unexpected frost, transplant your basil plant to a pot and bring it indoors to a south-facing window until the threat of frost as passed. Basil typically only grows in USDA zones 9 and above.

To Preserve

Basil is best preserved frozen in oil or infused in oil or vinegar and then jarred. Basil leaves can also be dried (though this can be a bit difficult) by hanging small bunches upside down a warm, dry place for a couple weeks.

Herbal Spotlight

Did you know that the flavor of basil intensifies when it is cooked? It's true! Unlike many other herbs, cooked basil leaves will have a stronger, more potent taste than fresh leaves from the same plant.

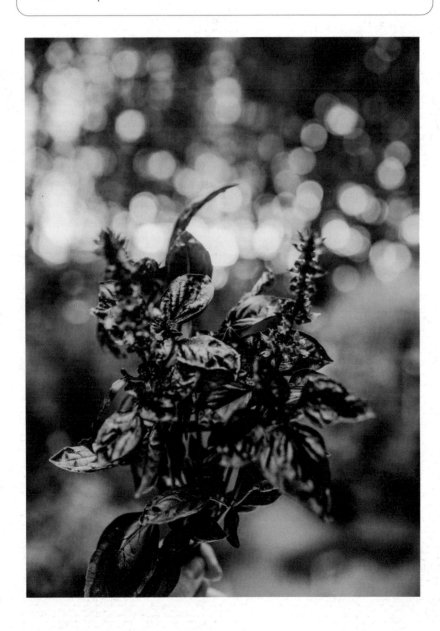

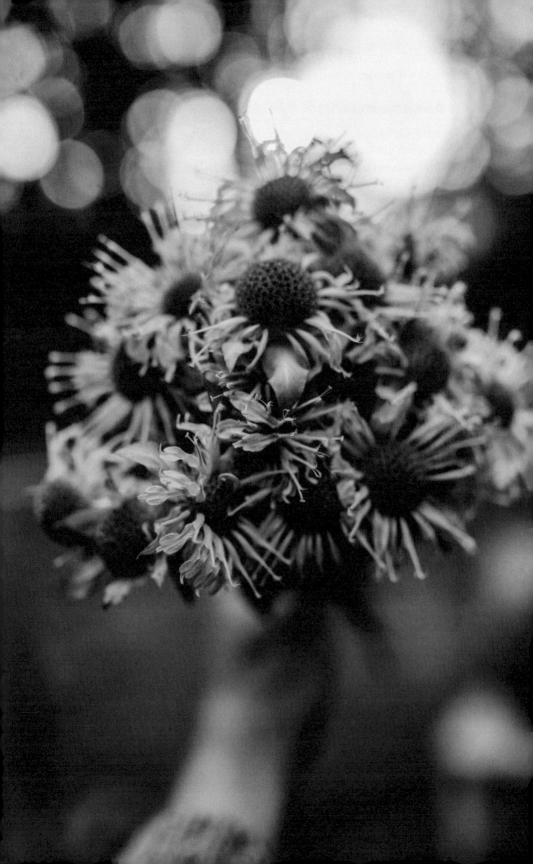

Bee Balm *Monarda spp.*

"...since plants are medicines,
so too could their stories be healing."

—*Robin Wall Kimmerer*, *Braiding Sweetgrass*

A member of the Lamiaceae (mint) family, this incredibly fragrant and beautiful herb is one of my very favorite perennials to grow in my garden due to its medicinal properties, delectable minty-citrus aroma, and vibrant colors. There are many varieties of bee balm available, with thistle-like flowers in shades of pink, red, and purple. The name, bee balm, is derived from its attractiveness to bees and other pollinators, but it is sometimes also referred to as bergamot (a nod to the bergamot orange), wild bergamot, crimson bee balm, scarlet Monarda, sweet leaf, Oswego tea, lemon mint, wound healer, or horsemint. In some parts of the world, it can grow wild and be foraged through the summer months. I consider bee balm a staple in every cottage, cut flower, and apothecary garden.

123

Beneficial Properties and Common Uses

Bee balm has many beneficial attributes, including antibacterial, antifungal, and anti-nausea properties used to naturally support those with eczema, sore throats, cold sores, achy muscles, and congestion. As a diaphoretic, it is used to naturally aid in relieving fevers. Fresh leaves can also be chewed as a natural mouthwash.

In the garden, bee balm attracts beneficial pollinators including bees, butterflies, and hummingbirds. I love having it readily available in my own backyard garden in case I cut or scratch myself while working in my garden. I simply tear a small portion of the stem off and apply the liquid inside directly to my scratch for instant cooling relief. Bee balm is a good garden companion for tomatoes, even improving their health and flavor.

In the kitchen, bee balm is the perfect addition to summer iced teas, lemonades, and cocktails. It is a wonderful substitute for mint, both muddled into the drink and as garnish, and is often used in hot teas and infusions as well. Added to salads, it gives greens a bold savory and minty boost. I most enjoy infusing honey with bee balm.

Around the home, fresh stalks can also be added to herbal shower bundles and are lovely, fragrant, and thoughtful additions to flower arrangements as a way to gift a beautiful and useful herb to someone you care about.

Try bee balm in the recipes and tutorials on pages 195, 198, 209, 221, 223, 231, 233, 235, 241, 262, 287

To Grow

To grow bee balm, start by selecting a location with full sun to partial shade and well-draining soil. Plant bee balm in the spring after the danger of frost has passed. I recommend planting two seeds in each hole, only about a quarter-inch deep. Then cover the top with a very light layer of soil. Be patient with bee balm, as it can take anywhere from ten to thirty days to germinate, but will be well worth the wait in the end. It is hardy in USDA zones 3–10.

Bee balm is a perennial and will grow up to three feet tall! Simply transplant it into your garden once the threat of frost has passed. When transplanting, keep in mind that the bee balm plant will grow larger each year. Because it self-seeds, bee balm can be considered a bit invasive, so a spacious garden bed or container is a good option. An organic fertilizer high in nitrogen and a big drink of water will help bee balm settle into its permanent living place in your garden, and pollinators will be forever grateful.

My favorite varieties of bee balm are Wild Bergamot, Scarlet Bee Balm, Monarda Beauty of Cobham, Monarda Balmy Lilac, and Monarda Balmy Pink.

Care and Harvest

Water the soil around the plants regularly, being careful not to overwater. Avoid getting the leaves or flowers wet. Deadhead spent blooms to encourage the growth of new flowers, and pinch back the stems to promote bushiness.

The best time of day to harvest bee balm is in the morning, after the dew has evaporated but before it gets too hot. This will ensure that you capture the greatest flavor and highest potency of medicinal properties. To harvest, cut the entire stalk when the small flowers have appeared (or even before). If you plan to use them fresh over the next few days, simply drop them into a vase of clean, cool water in your kitchen to enjoy their delicate beauty between uses.

Cut the entire plant back in the fall to prevent them from becoming too woody and to encourage new growth next year. Be sure to label the area to know where it will reemerge in the spring.

To Preserve

If you want to dry them, tie a few stalks together into a small bunch and hang upside down in a cool, dry, well-ventilated location for a few weeks. (I typically let mine hang for three weeks, and then check that the leaves crumble easily when pinched before breaking the flowers and leaves off the stems to jar.) Alternatively, you can use a dehydrator.

Herbal Spotlight
Bee balm leaves were used as a substitute for tea during the American Revolutionary War when black tea was scarce.

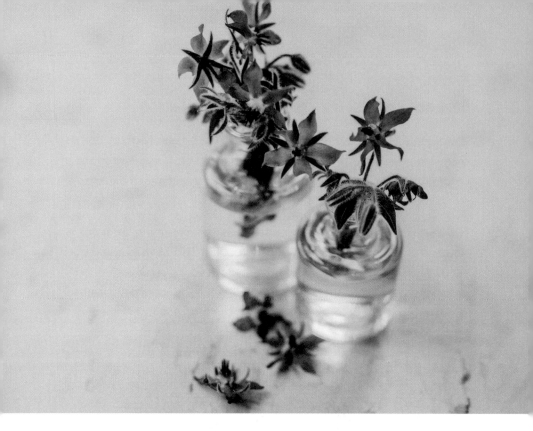

Borage *Borago officinalis*

"Borage always brings courage."

—*Pliny the Elder*. Roman author, naturalist,
and philosopher (AD 23–79)

Borage is an annual herb known for its delicate five-pointed, blue, star-shaped edible flowers. The leaves and flowers of the plant have a cucumber-like flavor and are commonly used in salads, soups, and drinks. There are several varieties of borage, including white-flowered and pink-flowered varieties, but the most common type, and my personal favorite, has blue star-shaped flowers. A single plant will produce hundreds of these gorgeous tiny flowers in a single season. Other common names for borage include starflower, bee bush, herb of gladness, burrage, borak, and bugloss.

Beneficial Properties and Common Uses

Borage has many beneficial attributes including anti-inflammatory and antioxidant properties used to naturally support those with rheumatoid arthritis, eczema, anxiety, respiratory issues, and fever. It can also be used to stimulate lactation in nursing mothers and is a common ingredient in skin-care products, used to soothe and moisturize skin. Borage is a rich source of essential fatty acids.

In the garden, borage attracts beneficial pollinators, including bees and butterflies. It is a good garden companion to tomatoes, squash, and strawberries.

I most enjoy using borage blossoms in the kitchen to garnish cocktails, iced summer drinks, infused waters, salads, and desserts, and to freeze inside ice cubes as a fun botanical detail.

> *Precautionary Note:* Borage is toxic to dogs, cats, and horses.

Try borage in the recipes and tutorials on pages 195, 198, 200, 215, 223, 249, 254, 269

To Grow

Borage is a relatively easy herb to grow and requires minimal care. It thrives in full sun and well-drained soil with a pH in the 6.0 to 7.0 range, but can tolerate a range of soil types. If starting from seed, sow directly into the ground in the spring or early summer, once all threat of frost has passed and soil has warmed a bit. (Borage can also be started indoors and then transplanted outside once the seedlings are established.) Sow two seeds into half-inch holes, and be sure to completely cover with soil, as they need darkness to germinate. Germination takes one to two weeks. Thin the seedlings as necessary once they're eight inches tall or have grown two sets of true leaves. Borage grows quickly and can become quite tall, so it needs plenty of room to grow. Even though it's technically considered an annual, it self-seeds easily, so once you've incorporated it into your garden, it's likely it will return year after year.

Alternatively, starter plants can be purchased from your local garden center and planted out two weeks after the last frost, when the soil and air temperatures are beginning to warm. Borage grows in USDA zones 3–10, blooming from early summer often through to the first frost.

Care and Harvest

Water regularly, but try not to overwater, as borage prefers a slightly drier soil. To harvest, simply snip fresh leaves and flowers as needed with clean garden shears, but try to do so before leaves develop their rough bristly hairs. Flowers can be snipped individually or as entire clusters as soon as they've opened.

To Preserve

Borage is best enjoyed fresh; however, I love adding the flowers to my ice cube trays before freezing. Those gorgeous little flowers are the perfect size and smile up at you from your cool drink on summer days. Borage can also be pressed and used in botanical arts and crafts.

Herbal Spotlight
Borage flowers are not only edible, but are also used as a natural food dye to color icings, or beverages.

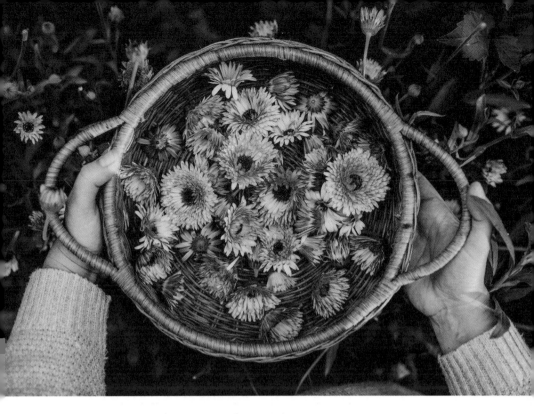

Calendula *Calendula officinalis*

"Calendula, the marigold, is a joy to the heart
and sight of the gardener and nature lover alike."

—*Maureen Rogers*, herbalist

Calendula is an annual herb known for its medicinal, culinary, and ornamental attributes. It is easy to grow and pollinator friendly. There are several varieties of calendula, including single-flowered and double-flowered varieties in varying shades of yellow and orange, and even some new varieties with pink hues. I consider calendula another staple in every cottage and apothecary garden. Calendula has other common names, including common marigold, prophetic marigold, Scottish marigold, Marybud, summer's bride, ruddles, and throughout-the-months.

Beneficial Properties and Common Uses

Calendula is most widely appreciated for its anti-inflammatory, antibacterial and antifungal properties, making it a popular choice for naturally healing cuts, scrapes, and scratches, and to naturally support those with dry skin, eczema, rashes, menstrual cramps, and digestive issues. Calendula is commonly infused in oil and used as a nourishing ingredient in skin-care products, including creams, lotions, balms, and salves, and is safe to be used topically on children.

> "Calendula strengthens the heart exceedingly."
>
> —*Nicholas Culpeper*, English botanist, herbalist, physician, and astrologer (1616-1654)

In the garden, calendula is a natural pest repellant and an excellent garden companion to tomatoes and carrots. Its vibrant colors attract beneficial pollinators, including bees and butterflies.

Around the home, calendula can be used as a natural food coloring and has beautiful ornamental properties, making it a lovely addition to cut-flower arrangements.

My favorite varieties of calendula are Sunset Buff (sometimes called Bronze Beauty), Pink Surprise (sometimes called Peach Surprise), Ivory Princess, Peach Apricot Beauty, and Zeolights.

Try calendula in the recipes and tutorials on pages 196, 209, 215, 223, 233, 235, 241, 254, 259, 262, 270, 279, 287

To Grow

Calendula is a beautiful and versatile herb that is easy to grow. Start by selecting a sunny location in your growing space with rich, well-draining soil. Calendula seeds can be sown directly into the soil in the early spring, or you can start them indoors four to six weeks before the last frost date. If starting indoors, I recommend planting one or two seeds in each hole, about a half-inch deep and eight inches apart, and covering the hole with soil. They usually germinate in just two to three days on heat (six to nine days with no heat mat). Once your seedlings begin to grow, make sure to water them regularly and keep the soil moist but not waterlogged. Calendula lives happily in the ground, in garden beds, or in smaller containers. It can reach up to fifteen inches tall.

Alternatively, starter plants can be purchased from your local garden center and planted out two weeks after the last frost, when the soil and air temperatures are beginning to warm. Calendula grows in USDA zones 3–10.

Care and Harvest

Be careful not to overwater calendula, and deadhead the spent blooms regularly to encourage more flowering. Fertilize once a month with an organic balanced fertilizer.

Harvest calendula in the morning, when possible, after dew has dried off but before temperatures rise. You will notice that calendula flowers close up overnight and open again with the sun. Ideally, you want to harvest when the blooms are half-open (or just opened that day) and dry, with no drops of water or dew. If harvesting for flower arrangements, cut the entire stem. If harvesting for medicinal or culinary purposes, pinch the flower at the base of the head with your finger and thumb or snip with clean shears. (I prefer to use snips because calendula can leave a sticky residue on skin.) If using fresh, remove the petals from the center, as the center can be very bitter. Harvesting early and often (at least once a week) will encourage continued blooms and bountiful harvests long into the final days of summer. Calendula is an annual and will need to be planted again each year.

To Preserve

To dry calendula, spread them over a screen or basket that allows airflow and circulation around it. Shake or flip the flowers every few days so all sides dry evenly. The length of time necessary to dry this flower depends greatly on its size and the temperature and moisture of the space you're drying it in. Start with three weeks, and then check to ensure they are brittle and dry before storing the heads whole in a clean, dry glass jar tightly closed with a lid until you're ready to use them. Alternatively, you can use a dehydrator. Calendula can be pressed and used in botanical arts and crafts.

Herbal Spotlight

Calendula is sometimes called the "herb of the sun" because its flowers open and close with the sun and follow the sun's movement throughout the day, from east to west. This phenomenon is known as *heliotropism*, rooted in ancient Greek *helio* referring to "sun," and "tropism" referring to the turning of a living organism toward (or away) from an external stimulus, which is, in this case, light.

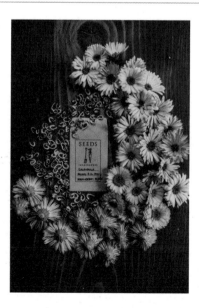

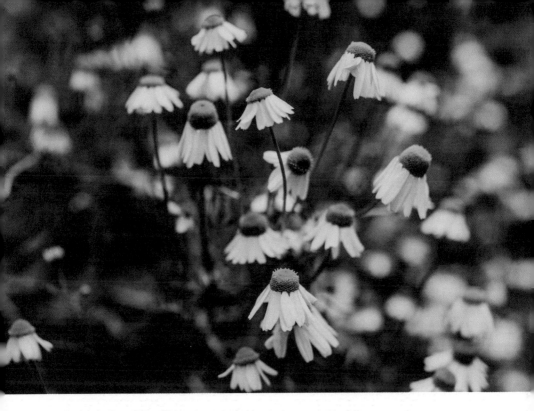

Chamomile *Matricaria chamomilla*

"Chamomile, the more it is trodden on, the faster it grows, spreading its sweet scent around the garden."

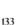

—*Mary Elizabeth Braddon*, English novelist (1835–1915)

Hands down, my favorite herbal fragrance in my garden is the sweet, fruity aroma of chamomile. A member of the Asteraceae family, chamomile refers to two different plants, Roman chamomile and German chamomile. Both are tall-growing annual varieties that produce dainty daisy-like flowers with yellow centers and white petals. It has long been used in teas and considered a "healing herb," valued for its many beneficial properties. Chamomile is sometimes referred to as wild chamomile, blue chamomile, true chamomile, or scented mayweed. It is easy to grow, prolific, and very pollinator friendly, making it a fantastic choice for every garden.

Beneficial Properties and Common Uses

Chamomile is prized for its soothing and nourishing properties, but also has anti-inflammatory and antibacterial properties that naturally support those suffering from bloating, cramping, and indigestion. It is also sometimes used as a mild sedative to calm nerves, promote relaxation, and improve sleep quality and is used to naturally support those with anxiety, stress, and depression. It is commonly incorporated into iced and hot herbal teas or infused into oils and commonly used in various skin-care products such as balms, lotions, and salves for its medicinal properties and lovely fragrance.

In the garden, it is easy to grow, fragrant, and attracts many beneficial pollinators such as bees and butterflies. It is also known to deter mosquitoes. It is a good garden-bed companion to cabbage and onions, even improving their growth and flavor.

Around the home, chamomile can be used as a natural dye and makes a lovely fragrant filler for cut-flower arrangements. I love dropping a fistful of chamomile stems into a vase of cold water and placing it next to my bathroom sink to enjoy the light, breezy fragrance every time I walk by.

Try chamomile in the recipes and tutorials on pages 195, 198, 209, 215, 231, 233, 235, 241, 259, 262, 279, 287

To Grow

Sow chamomile seeds directly in the soil in late fall, after the first killing frost, by broadcast-sowing it (sprinkling evenly across) over moistened soil. Press them firmly into the soil, but do not cover them. This process allows the seeds to naturally cold-stratify.

If you prefer to grow chamomile in the spring, I recommend starting indoors about six weeks before your zone's last frost date. I prefer to broadcast-sow the seeds into containers that I can simply pick up and relocate to the garden once it warms up. I've found this transplant system easier than transplanting out several small bunches in smaller seed-starting pots. Chamomile needs light to germinate, so do not cover the seeds with soil, but do press them firmly into your moistened soil and put them under grow lights right away. Use a misting can or water bottle to sprinkle water very gently over the top of the seeds from an arm's length above, so the mist falls onto the seeds without blowing them away. There is no need to bottom-water this seed. Germination typically occurs in ten to fourteen days.

Chamomile thrives in a sunny location with rich, organic, well-draining soil and is happy in the ground, in a garden bed, or in a container. However, if you live in a hot climate, I recommend planting chamomile in a container that you can easily move into partial shade if you see that your plant is looking stressed. Chamomile is hardy in USDA zones 3–9.

Alternatively, starter plants are often available at your local garden center and should be planted out after your zone's last frost date.

My Favorite Varieties

- **Zloty Lan** (*Matricaria recutita*)—Polish variety, bigger and higher-yielding, wonderful choice for all medicinal and culinary purposes
- **Roman** (*Anthemis nobilis*)—most commonly used in potpourri, teas, cosmetics, and skin-care products; less bitter than German
- **German** (*Matricaria recutita*) most common in teas

Care and Harvest

Chamomile needs consistent moisture to grow well, so make sure to water your plants regularly. If you're growing chamomile in a pot, just make sure it has plenty of drainage holes to prevent waterlogging. Be careful not to overwater, as this can cause the roots to rot. Chamomile resents being transplanted after its first bloom, so keep this in mind when choosing a growing container.

Chamomile flowers are ready to be harvested when fully opened. Gently pop the flower heads off the stem, using your thumb and index finger, or cut them with a clean pair of garden snips. The leaves can also be harvested.

To Preserve

Chamomile is a great candidate for drying. Simply scatter the collected flower heads on a screen to dry in a warm, dry place, or use a dehydrator. Once dry, store them in an airtight glass container for up to one year. Chamomile can also be pressed and used in botanical arts and crafts.

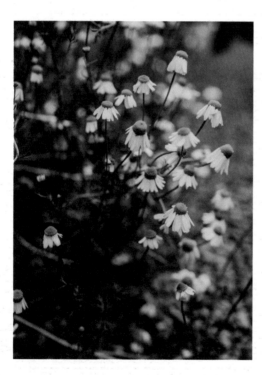

Herbal Spotlight
Did you know that chamomile has a long history of use in the brewing of beer? In medieval Europe, chamomile was often used as a flavoring agent in beer and was believed to have a preservative effect that helped to extend the shelf life of the beer. Today, chamomile is still used by some craft brewers as a unique and flavorful ingredient in their recipes.

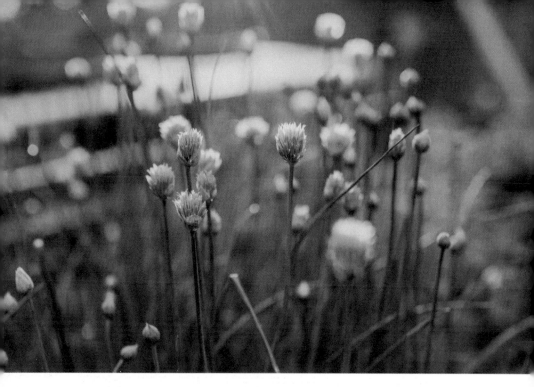

Chive *Allium schoenoprasum*

"Onion is a humble vegetable, but it has saved
countless recipes from mediocrity. Its flavor
and aroma can transform the ordinary into
the extraordinary."

—*Yotam Ottolenghi*, British chef and food writer

Belonging to the onion family, chive is a kitchen-friendly perennial
herb with countless culinary uses. It has long, thin, green leaves that
grow twelve inches tall and are hollow and tubular in shape, growing in
clumps. They grow lavender-colored blossoms that are also edible. It
is known for its delicate and slightly sweet, sometimes garlicky, flavor.
Chives are easy to grow and one of the first greens to pop up in my
spring garden. Chives are sometimes referred to as sweth or rush leeks.

Beneficial Properties and Common Uses

Chive has many beneficial properties, including being rich in vitamin C, K, and A, and in minerals including calcium, phosphorus, and potassium. It is used to naturally detoxify the body, boost skin health, lower blood pressure, and regulate cholesterol.

Most commonly used in the kitchen, chives are often minced and sprinkled fresh atop soups, salads, biscuits, baked potato, omelets, scrambles, and other egg dishes, or whipped into cream cheese, dressings, dips, or compound butter. I most enjoy creating a finishing salt with them. Even the pretty blossoms are edible, making a gorgeous, colorful, and flavorful vinegar or a beautiful pop of color, texture, and flavor atop salads.

In the garden, chive is prized as an easy-to-grow perennial with a long growing season, even year-round in some climates. It attracts pollinators, including bees and butterflies, while repelling garden pests like aphids and Japanese beetles. Chive is naturally deer- and rabbit-resistant and a good companion to roses, tomatoes, carrots, and strawberries.

138

Try chive in the recipes and tutorials on pages 190, 192, 195, 221, 223, 235, 242, 270

To Grow

If direct-seeding, wait until after your zone's last frost date. Chives prefer fertile, loamy soil. If starting indoors, you can broadcast-sow chive seeds any time of the year and successfully grow them indoors or transplant them out once the threat of frost has passed. Broadcast-sow chive seeds over dampened soil. Press them firmly into the soil but do not cover them, as they require light to germinate. Water carefully with a misting can or bottom-water until germination occurs. You can expect germination in ten to fourteen days. Chives are hardy in USDA zones 3–10.

Alternatively, starter plants are often available at your local garden center and should be planted out after your zone's last frost date.

Care and Harvest

Chives thrive in bright sunny growing spaces, but can also tolerate partial shade. They are happiest in pots and containers, though I also grow them successfully in the corners of my garden beds. Be careful not to overfertilize, as it will weaken their flavor. (I prefer not to fertilize my chives at all.)

When chives grow to be about twelve inches tall, gather a handful of the tubular leaves in one hand and snip with clean kitchen shears about three-quarters of the way down the plant. Choose ones that have the boldest greenish-blue color for the best flavor and scent. Remove any that are wilting or yellowing along the way. Collect the chive blossoms as well, which are also edible; however, the stalk of the blossom is typically too tough and less flavorful, so I clip the blossom off and compost the stalk.

In the fall, you can divide your chives and bring some inside to continue to grow all winter long, or cut them to the ground and label the area, so you know where to expect them to reemerge next spring.

139

To Preserve

Chives can be dried, but I do feel they lose some of their flavor when preserving them this way. To dry chives, cut them into very small pieces with your kitchen shears and then lay them flat on a cookie sheet lined with parchment paper and bake for an hour at 200 degrees Fahrenheit, stirring them from time to time. Let them cool completely before storing in an airtight glass container for up to one year. Alternatively, chives dry well in a dehydrator. Chives can also be infused in oils and vinegars. Lastly, you can fill ice cube trays with chives and then water to freeze them into cubes for individual use throughout the year. I have found that this changes the texture of the herbs and decreases flavor.

Herbal Spotlight
In the early 1900s, *chive* was a slang word meaning "a shout."

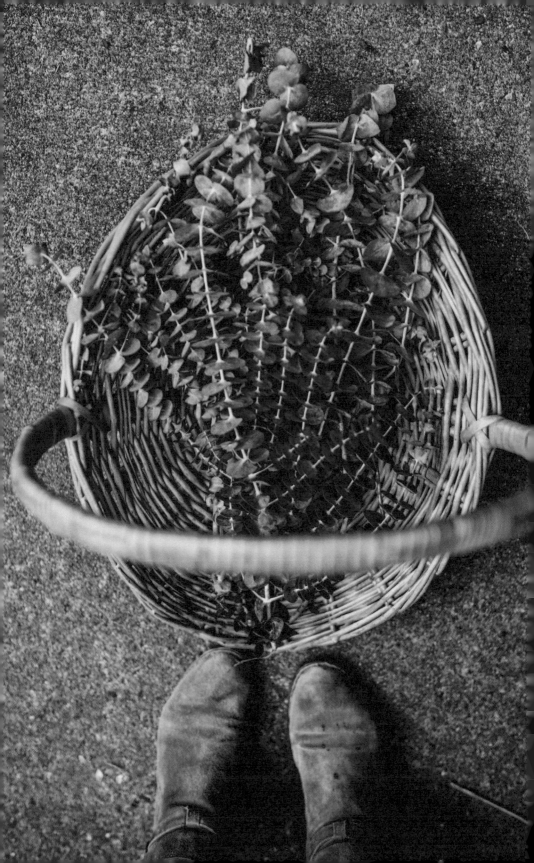

Eucalyptus *Eucalyptus spp.*

"All that man needs for health
and healing has been provided by God in nature,
the challenge of science is to find it."

—*Paracelsus* (1493–1541)

A member of the Myrtaceae family, eucalyptus is actually a genus of tree and shrub but, due to its many medicinal attributes, it is often categorized as an herb and included in many herbal recipes. While there are over seven hundred species of eucalyptus, *Eucalyptus globulus* is most often used in herbalism. Eucalyptus is known for its strongly scented blue-green foliage which produces essential oil that is commonly used in aromatherapy. It is sometimes referred to as blue gum, southern blue gum, Tasmanian blue gum, Tasmanian oak, Victorian blue gum, gum tree, or fever tree.

Beneficial Properties and Common Uses

One of my favorite plants in my garden is eucalyptus, for its aromatic scent commonly thought to have a calming effect and often used in aromatherapy. It has many beneficial attributes as well, including anti-inflammatory, astringent, antimicrobial, and antiseptic properties used to naturally treat cuts and scratches and support those with sinus congestion, sore throats, sore joints and muscles, colds and flus, and respiratory ailments including asthma, bronchitis, and cough.

In the garden, eucalyptus acts as a pest repellant, as most insects do not like its scent.

Around the home, eucalyptus is a common ingredient in household cleaning products, air fresheners, and insect repellents, and is a beautiful and fragrant addition to floral arrangements and wreaths. It can also be added to fresh botanical shower bundles and steamers.

Silver bell caps can be used as a natural button and are gorgeous seasonal additions to floral arrangements, wreaths, and other crafting projects.

> *Precautionary Note:* Fresh eucalyptus leaves are toxic if consumed, so never ingest them. Eucalyptus oil is also toxic when ingested.

Try eucalyptus in the recipes and tutorials on pages 202, 209, 231, 233, 235, 256, 261, 262, 279, 283, 285, 287

To Grow

Eucalyptus thrives in cool, wet winters and dry, hot summers, and requires plenty of sunlight and well-drained soil. Start indoors ten to twelve weeks prior to your zone's last frost date. Sow seeds on the surface of moistened soil but do not cover, as eucalyptus needs light to germinate. Use a misting can or water bottle to sprinkle water very gently over top of the seeds from an arm's length above, so the mist falls onto the seeds without blowing them away. After sprouts appear, bottom-watering is sufficient. Germination takes an average of forty-five days. While it is very slow to germinate, once established, eucalyptus will quickly become one of the fastest-growing plants in your garden. (I start my eucalyptus from seed in January.) It will need to be pruned regularly to control its size and shape. Eucalyptus typically grows in USDA zones 8–11. For climates that dip below 50 degrees Fahrenheit during the cold months, I recommend growing eucalyptus in containers and overwintering them, bringing the containers inside when temperatures drop, and then returning them outside when it warms again in the spring.

Alternatively, they can be purchased as starter plants and planted out after your zone's last frost date.

My favorite varieties of eucalyptus are Silver Dollar, Baby Blue, and Round-Leaved Mallee.

Care and Harvest

The branches should be harvested when they are mature but prior to flowering, by clipping them with clean pruning shears. If using in floral arrangements, condition each stem by removing the leaves on the bottom two-thirds to ensure that no leaves are submerged in water. They have a two-week (often more) vase life.

To Preserve

Air-dry the leaves on a screen in a cool place, out of direct sunlight, or hang upside down in small bunches. Once fully dried, store leaves in an airtight glass container for up to one year. Eucalyptus can also be pressed and used in botanical arts and crafts.

Herbal Spotlight

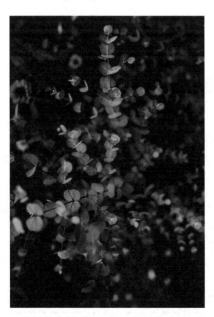

Did you know that the roots of all species of eucalyptus release a toxic chemical that inhibits the growth of any plants sharing the same soil around it? It's true, so be careful where you plant them! I have given all my eucalyptus plants their own dedicated containers and recommend doing this so you can easily relocate them indoors if you experience harsh winters or unusual dips in temperature.

143

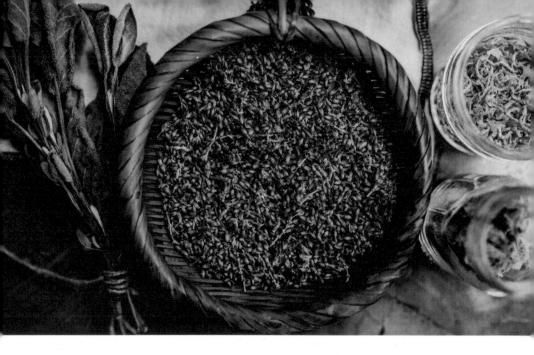

Lavender *Lavandula angustifolia*

> "The air was fragrant with a thousand trodden aromatic herbs, with fields of lavender, and with the brightest roses blushing in tufts all over the meadows."
>
> —*William C. Bryant,* American poet and writer (1794–1878)

A member of the Lamiaceae (mint) family, lavender is a perennial evergreen shrub best known for its sweet, calming, and uplifting fragrance. A staple in cottage gardens around the world, the lavender plant is easy to maintain, drought-tolerant, and thrives in many climates. This beautiful and heavenly-scented herb holds a special place in my family's heart. We have planted lavender near the front entrance of every home we've ever owned and have fond memories of family trips to Washington's incredible lavender fields, where our children would run the purple rows and mazes for hours. Lavender has woody branches with upright, straight, leafy, green spikey shoots. The leaves are a beautiful cool-toned gray-green color with small, dark purple (or sometimes violet, white, or pink) flowers on the tips that give the herb its heavenly scent. It can grow up to three feet tall; however, most shrubs are closer to twenty-four inches. English lavender is the most common species used for culinary and medicinal purposes and is my personal favorite as well.

Beneficial Properties and Common Uses

Lavender is one of my favorite herbs for its numerous beneficial attributes, including antibacterial and antiseptic properties; it can be used to naturally disinfect cuts and reduce scarring. It can also be used to naturally support those with insect bites and stings, eczema, burns, and sore muscles. Its calming and soothing mild sedative properties can be used to naturally relieve headaches, calm the mind, aid in a peaceful night of sleep, and relieve symptoms associated with anxiety and depression. Lavender aromatherapy is often used to naturally support those with Alzheimer's and dementia, and to help relieve stress, anxiety, sleeplessness, hypertension, headaches, pre-eclampsia, constipation, labor pain, postnatal healing, and post-partum depression in pregnant women. It is most commonly infused into oils and used topically. Lavender essential oil is so useful that it is often called the "Swiss Army Knife of Essential Oils."

145

In the garden, lavender attracts beneficial insects, including bees, butterflies, and others. Additionally, it naturally repels flies, mosquitoes, and moths, and effectively kills lice and parasites.

In the kitchen, I most often use lavender to make simple syrups, garnish cocktails, and incorporate into lemonades and other iced drinks. It is also a lovely addition to hot teas, baked goods, and ice cream. English lavender is also one of the herbs in the spice blend called *herbes de Provence*.

Around the home, lavender water is used as a linen and pillow spray, and lavender essential oil is a common ingredient in homemade deodorants. The essential oil of lavender can be added to diffusers for its aromatherapy benefits, and it is generally safe to be used on children. Dried lavender buds can be collected in sachets and tucked under pillows or in clothing drawers. Its ornamental properties can also be appreciated as a wreath hung in the home or on a door, inviting visitors in with its lovely color and fragrance.

Try lavender in the recipes and tutorials on pages 195, 196, 198, 204, 209, 215, 221, 226, 231, 233, 235, 237, 241, 249, 252, 254, 256, 262, 269, 270, 279, 287

To Grow

Because growing lavender from seed is rather difficult, I recommend purchasing lavender as a small shrub from your local nursery. (If you wish to grow it from seed, keep in mind that lavender seed needs light to germinate, and germination may take a month or more.) Space lavender plants twelve to eighteen inches apart, in an area with plenty of sunlight and sandy (even rocky) soil that has a pH of 6.7 to 7.3. If the shrub is small, mix some compost into the soil to give it a jump start. Once established, lavender is easy to maintain and very rewarding. It grows well in the ground, in garden beds, or in pots. Most varieties of English lavender are hardy in USDA zones 5–9. Spanish lavender is only hardy in zones 7–9 and French lavender in zones 8–11.

Lavender is relatively easy to grow from cuttings. Learn more about the propagation process on page 93.

I prefer to grow English lavender, which has a much stronger fragrance than Spanish lavender, and a much sweeter fragrance than French lavender, which has more pine notes. There are many lovely and aromatic varieties of English lavender to choose from, but my favorites are Hidcote, Munstead, Betty's Blue, Grosso, Beuna Vista, Impress Purple, and Royal Purple. For a white lavender, try Edelweiss, Melissa, or Jean Davis. For Spanish lavender, try Ballerina, Madrid Purple, or Curly Top.

Care and Harvest

While lavender does not like to be watered frequently, it is important to water it deeply every few weeks during the hottest seasons of the year.

Harvest lavender in the morning after dew has evaporated from the buds, keeping in mind that only the flowers of lavender are harvested. Always harvest flower buds when the buds show their deep bright color, but before they open. Gather a handful of sprigs below the flowers in one hand, and cut underneath your hand, just above the leaves or side branches, with clean pruning snips or kitchen shears. Once the flowers are removed, the plant will begin to redirect its energy to new growth. Never cut the woody part of the stem. Choose a completely dry day, and dry your flower buds as soon as possible after harvesting to decrease the likelihood of molding. Do not expose the buds to heat, which can lessen their essential oils and lovely aroma.

To Preserve

Air-dry lavender sprigs on a screen in a cool place, out of direct sunlight, or bundle them tightly into small bundles and hang upside down until the buds are brittle and easily fall off (about two weeks). Alternatively, a dehydrator can be used. Once fully dried and brittle, the buds will easily fall off the stems when rolled lightly between your fingers. Store the buds in an airtight glass container. Every time you open it, it will be like a rush of summer flowing out of the jar. Or lavender buds can be left on their stems after drying and added to preserved flower arrangements or wreaths. Lavender can also be infused in oil or water, steeped into a simple syrup, frozen into ice cubes, or pressed and used in botanical arts and crafts.

147

Herbal Spotlight
Lavender was used as a secret ingredient in Coca-Cola in the 1930s! The company used lavender oil as a flavoring in the popular soda, along with other ingredients such as vanilla, cinnamon, and citrus oils. While lavender was eventually removed from the recipe, it's still an interesting bit of trivia about the history of this beloved plant.

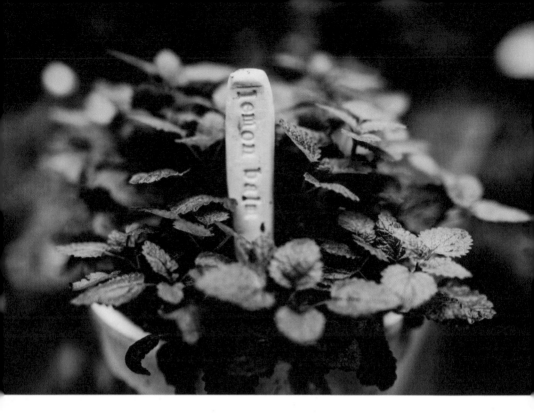

Lemon Balm *Melissa officinalis*

"Lemon balm causeth the heart and mind
to become merry."

—*Avicenna*, physician and philosopher (970–1037)

I am a huge fan of lemon balm and am on a personal mission to inspire everyone to grow and use it. A member of the Lamiaceae (mint) family, lemon balm has vibrant green heart-shaped leaves with toothed margins and a bright lemony scent and flavor. Lemon balm is sometimes called sweet balm, sweet Mary, Melissa, balm mint, blue balm, gentle balm, honey leaf, honey plant, or heart's delight. It is one of my very favorite perennials in my garden, and I find myself dividing my plants every year to grow more.

Beneficial Properties and Common Uses

Rich in vitamins and minerals, lemon balm has many beneficial attributes, including antimicrobial, antiviral, and mild antidepressant properties which can be used to naturally support those with headaches, digestive issues, nausea, abdominal paint, menstrual cramps, anxiety, and mild depression when ingested as an herbal tea or used in aromatherapy. When used topically, it naturally supports those with bee and wasp stings and skin conditions such as ulcers, wounds, scratches, scrapes, and cold sores. As a gentle nervine, it is safe to use on children. It can be infused in honey and used as a calming nighttime syrup to calm and rejuvenate the nervous system and promote peaceful sleep in both children and adults. Lemon balm is used to naturally improve memory and concentration and is used to support those with Alzheimer's disease and attention-deficit hyperactivity disorder (ADHD).

In the garden, lemon balm is a natural insect repellant, protecting your crops from garden pests, and is deer- and rabbit-resistant. I recommend distributing it throughout your entire garden and placing pots of it near outdoor seating and dining areas, but keep in mind that your plant will grow bushier each year.

In the kitchen, lemon balm can be used to make a delicious and refreshing batch of lemonade or added to other iced drinks. I most enjoy using lemon balm as a garnish for cocktails and salads, and making candied lemon balm chips and decorating cookies with them.

Around the home, lemon balm is a rejuvenating addition to herbal bath bundles and bath soaks, and makes a fragrant addition to floral arrangements. It can also be used to make natural mosquito repellant sprays.

> *Precautionary Note:* Lemon balm has been known to lower thyroid levels, so refrain from using it if you have thyroid disease.

Try lemon balm in the recipes and tutorials on pages 190, 195, 196, 198, 217, 221, 226, 231, 233, 235, 241, 269, 270, 273

To Grow

Lemon balm loves dappled sunlight and moist but well-drained soil. It is very easy to grow from seed, either directly sown into the ground after all threat of frost has passed, or started indoors six to eight weeks prior to your zone's last frost date. It grows rapidly outdoors and can also be grown successfully indoors in containers. I recommend pots or other preferred type of container rather than a seed tray for this particular plant, as they are broadcast instead of individually sown. To sow lemon balm seeds, simply sprinkle them evenly across your container or pot. Do not cover, as they need light to germinate. A heat mat will expedite the germination process, which should take about a week. Lemon balm is hardy in USDA zones 4–9 and will thrive in most gardens.

Alternatively, starter plants are often available at your local garden center and should be planted out after your zone's last frost date.

Lemon balm is also easy to grow from cuttings. Learn more about the propagation method on page 93.

Care and Harvest

Lemon balm is best harvested in the morning, when the leaves are their most potent and dry, but before the plant flowers. Use clean garden shears or snips to cut the stems about six inches above the base, which ensures regrowth of the herb. In most conditions, lemon balm can easily be cut two to three times in a season. The more you cut, the more it will grow! Deep intermittent watering is preferred over light watering every day. Always water the soil underneath the plant, rather than pouring water over the foliage.

Lemon balm can easily be divided (a process called root division) by carefully breaking the entire plant in half, separating the root system, and then transplanting the segmented clumps into different areas, which will each continue to multiply over time. I recommend dividing the plant every few years.

At the end of the growing season, cut your lemon balm plant back to an inch above the ground. Be sure to label the location so you know where it will reemerge next spring. If you grow lemon balm in a container that can be moved, simply relocate it into your greenhouse or to a south-facing windowsill in your home to enjoy its bright lemony fragrance on even the coldest winter days.

To Preserve

Fresh leaves will begin to discolor if touched too often, and since lemon balm can be grown indoors year-round, I recommend using it fresh. However, it can be dried if processed carefully, handling the leaves as minimally as possible. Spread in a single layer on drying screens to ensure constant airflow. I even run a fan in the room where I'm drying lemon balm. Alternatively, you can cut further down the stem and then tie small bundles of balm tightly and hang them upside down. Avoid light exposure during the drying process, and dry at low temperatures of around 86 degrees Fahrenheit. Lemon balm can also be pressed and used in botanical arts and crafts.

151

Herbal Spotlight
Did you know that older, more mature lemon balm leaves have a stronger, more pungent flavor than younger ones? So, as difficult as it is, avoid cutting the leaves too early!

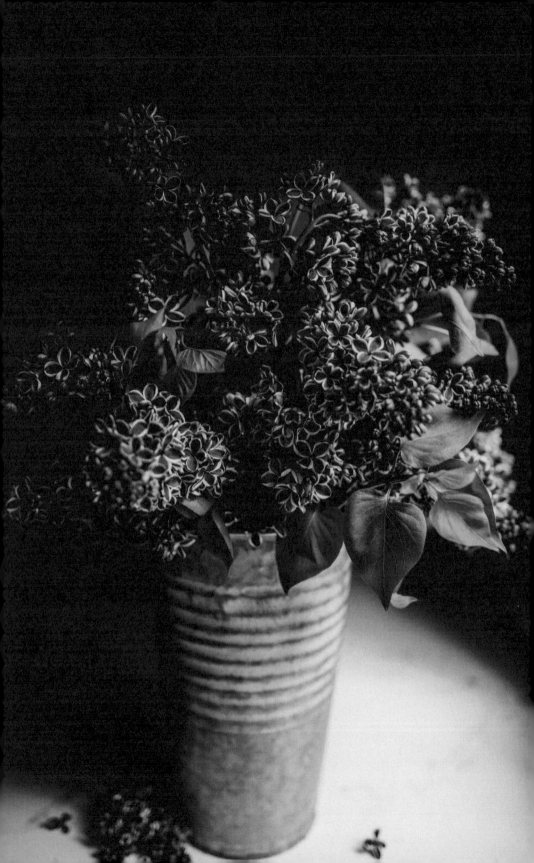

Lilac *Syringa culfaris*

"The smell of moist earth and lilacs hung in the air like wisps of the past and hints of the future."

—*Margaret Millar*, American Canadian writer (1915–1994)

A member of the Oleaceae (olive) family, lilac is an amazing and beautiful perennial shrub or tree that blooms in late April or early May. While there is some debate surrounding its categorization in the botanical world, for the sake of this book and due to its abundance of medicinal qualities, we will consider lilac an herb, as it has been considered in Eastern Europe and Asia for thousands of years. Lilac is a deciduous, multi-stemmed upright shrub with strong stems and dark green heart-shaped leaves. With its broad, pointed clusters of small fragrant flowers ranging in color from light to dark purple hues to shades of pink, blue, magenta, or even white or yellow, lilac really is a show for the senses! Some varieties, like Peking and Japanese, can reach heights of up to thirty feet! Lilacs can live to be well over a hundred years old, often outliving the gardener who planted them and the architecture they were planted near.

153

Beneficial Properties and Common Uses

Lilac has an abundance of beneficial properties, in the blossoms as well as the bark of the plant. The blossoms are a natural antiseptic, preventing the growth of bacteria, and have antiviral and antimicrobial properties. They are often used to relieve cough and congestion, and aid in digestion. Their anticoagulant properties help thin blood and prevent clotting, while their purgative properties simultaneously expel toxins from the body. Lilac bark is perhaps most often used to reduce fevers but is often recognized in the skin-care field as an astringent, tightening soft tissue and toning skin. The bark also acts as an anti-inflammatory and can help reduce swelling in the body and remove toxins from the blood.

In the garden, lilac is prized for its ornamental characteristics and heavenly scent. The most recognized variety for fragrance is the Chinese lilac (*Syringa pubescens*), which has the ability to infuse entire outdoor gardens with its beautiful aroma. Lilac is also pollinator friendly, attracting butterflies, hummingbirds, and bees, among many other pollinators. Additionally, lilac shrubs and trees provide a protective nesting habitat for birds. These birds make homes in the lilac bushes and feast on the nearby insects, acting as a natural pest control for your garden space.

In the kitchen, all types of lilac blossoms are edible and are often used fresh to garnish salads, to decorate baked goods, and infused in hot or iced teas. I use lilac blossoms to make lilac simple syrups and cordials, to decorate cakes and cookies, and frozen into ice cubes to add botanical flair and a light floral taste to cold drinks.

When planted strategically near your home, lilac bushes can be good sources of privacy and shade.

Try lilac in the recipes and tutorials on pages 195, 198, 209, 215, 221, 231, 235, 241

To Grow

Because germination of lilac seeds is generally low and difficult, I recommend purchasing lilac starter plants from your favorite local nursery. The best time to plant lilac bushes is in the early spring or early autumn. Choose a spot that receives a minimum of six hours of direct sunlight daily during the spring and summer months, and with well-draining soil rich in organic matter. Break the soil up and supplement it with organic compost as necessary. Dig a hole that is deeper and wider than the container the lilac came in, carefully remove the root base from the container, and gently loosen the roots. Place the root ball in the hole and backfill it with soil, tamping down as you go. Mound the excess soil slightly around the base of the plant and then cover with mulch. Finally, give your new lilac a big drink of water. If you are planting multiple lilacs at one time, give them plenty of space to spread out, leaving approximately five feet of space between them, even if you are planting them to act as privacy hedges. USDA zones 3–8 are ideal for growing lilacs, though some varieties are cold hardy in zone 2.

Care and Harvest

Lilacs are considered a low-maintenance plant that require minimal care other than an occasional pruning. Fertilizing once in the early spring will give blooms a jump start; however, make sure the organic fertilizer you choose has low amounts of nitrogen, as too much can result in insufficient flowering. Remove spent blooms regularly to encourage more blooms later. This is the only pruning that is needed until your bushes reach at least six feet tall. Once they reach six feet, the best time to prune is right after flowering has finished. This gives the plant plenty of time to reestablish new buds for next year. Using clippers, first cut off any branches that are growing close to the ground that may be sprouting off the main trunk. Then, remove approximately a third of the plant's stems at the base, including inner branches. This provides improved air circulation and gives all the remaining branches better access to sunlight.

To harvest lilac blooms, take a pair of sharp garden shears and a bucket of clean, cool water out with you. Look for clusters with at least 75 percent of their blooms open, as lilac blooms do not generally open more after they've been cut. Cut the stems six or so inches from the clusters and clip all foliage off the stem, so all hydration efforts go directly to the blossoms. If your branches have a woody stem, snip the bottom of the branch, parallel with the length of the branch, one inch up, and fray the ends a bit. Opening up woody stem ends allows

155

the stem to pull in more water and focus its efforts on hydrating the blossoms to extend the vase life of your beautiful blooms.

To Preserve

Air-dry lilac blossoms individually on a screen in a cool place, out of direct sunlight, or hang them individually upside down for about two weeks, or until the clusters are completely dry and brittle to the touch. Alternatively, a dehydrator can be used. Store the buds in an airtight glass container. Lilacs can also be infused in oil or water, steeped into a simple syrup, frozen into ice cubes, or pressed and used in botanical arts and crafts.

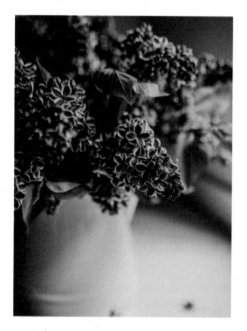

Herbal Spotlight
Did you know that purple and blue foods, like lilac, generally get their blueish hue from a flavonoid pigment called anthocyanin? This pigment contains large amounts of antioxidants, is thought to aid in the prevention of cardiovascular diseases, and has antidiabetic, anticancer, anti-inflammatory, antimicrobial, and even anti-obesity effects. Next time you pop a blue or purple herb in your mouth, feel confident you're doing your body good!

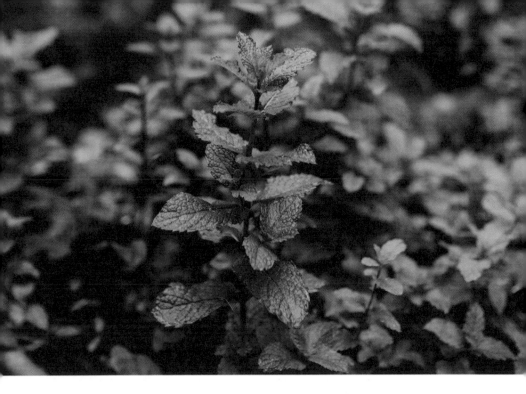

Mint *Mentha*

"The smell of mint, long celebrated for its restorative
properties, wafted through our kitchen, and
we knew that with mint came the possibility
of transformation."

—Ralph Waldo Emerson, American poet
and essayist (1803–1882)

There is nothing quite like the refreshing and invigorating scent of
freshly harvested mint and I couldn't imagine my garden without
several varieties of this gorgeous and useful perennial herb. A prolific
producer from early spring through first frost, it truly is a must-grow
for its culinary, medicinal, aromatherapy, and perfect addition to
floral arrangements. For the sake of simplicity, in this section, I have
compiled several similar varieties of mint (peppermint, spearmint,
doublemint, mountain mint, chocolate mint, lavender mint, mojito
mint, apple mint, and orange mint) under this all-encompassing
Mentha or "mint" category and section.

Beneficial Properties and Common Uses

Rich in vitamins and minerals, mint has a long list of beneficial attributes including antimicrobial, antiviral, antibacterial, antifungal, stimulating, relaxing, and dual warming and cooling properties that are well-known for naturally supporting those with digestive issues, headaches, toothaches, earaches, joint pain, muscle aches, respiratory congestion, anxiety, tension, nausea, motion sickness, and skin irritations including itchy skin, bug bites and rashes. As a natural stimulant, mint is often used to wake up, refresh, recharge, clear the mind, and increase concentration.

In the garden, mint attracts beneficial pollinators and insects and is a natural garden pest repellant. It is a good companion to tomatoes and cabbage, even improving their health and flavor.

In the kitchen, mint is most often used fresh as a popular culinary ingredient in drinks, salads, and desserts.

Around the home, mint is a common ingredient in mouthwashes, toothpaste, candy, gum, breath mints, lotions, and creams. I also love using mint as a flower arrangement filler.

Precautionary Note: Peppermint essential oil should always be diluted before use. Peppermint's high essential oil content makes it unsafe to use in high amounts during pregnancy or for babies and young children. Peppermint may reduce milk flow in nursing mothers. People with gastrointestinal reflux disease (GERD) may find that peppermint aggravates their condition. (Fresh or dried spearmint leaves, on the other hand, are particularly suited for children and pregnant women.)

Try mint in the recipes and tutorials on pages 195, 196, 198, 200, 202, 204, 210, 221, 223, 226, 231, 233, 235, 256, 262, 269, 277, 283, 285, 287

To Grow

I recommend starting mint indoors six to eight weeks prior to your zone's final frost date. Surface sow by gently pressing seeds into moistened soil then bottom water. Do not cover the seeds as they require light to germinate but a clear dome will help retain warmth. Germination will occur in 2 weeks, less with a heat mat. Once the seedlings are six inches tall, pinch the tops to promote a bushier plant shape and more branched stems. Mint is hardy in USDA zones 4-9 and will thrive in most gardens.

Alternatively, starter plants are often available at your local garden center and should be planted out after your zone's last frost date.

Mint is also easy to grow from cuttings. Learn more about the propagation method on page 93.

Care and Harvest

Mint is a vigorous perennial that will spread rampantly due to its incredibly strong underground root system, so careful consideration is necessary when deciding where to plant it. Since it can be a bit of a bully toward other plants around it and can easily overtake more vulnerable plants, I recommend dedicating a container to it alone. Whatever container you choose, make sure it is at least 18 inches deep and has several drainage holes.

Deep watering every week is all that is needed for mint. It is better to water less often for longer periods of time than to water lightly every day. Always water the soil underneath the plant rather than pouring water over the foliage. Harvest and prune mint often throughout the growing season. Harvest mint by cutting the top four to six inches of the stem just above a set of leaves.

My Favorite Varieties

- **Peppermint** (*Mentha piperita*) – probably the most popular of all the mints; known for its refreshing flavor and cooling sensation; common flavor in oral hygiene products and excellent floral arrangement filler

- **Spearmint** (*Mentha spicata*)—crisp but sweeter milder fragrance and flavor than peppermint with lighter green fuzzy foliage; excellent floral arrangement filler

- **Lavender Mint** (*Mentha piperita lavandula*)—deliciously floral overtones and a red stem; another excellent option for floral arrangements

- **Chocolate Mint** (*Mentha piperita f. citrata*)—unique flavor that combines the coolness of peppermint with a subtle chocolate taste; sometimes called peppermint patty mint; great for garnishing desserts

- **Orange Mint** (*Mentha piperita citrata*) stronger flavored than the other fruity mints; lovely notes of citrus and spice; also called Eau de Cologne mint or bergamot mint; excellent floral arrangement filler and used in salads, baked goods, simple syrups, and cocktails

To Preserve

Dry mint by spreading the foliage in a single layer on drying screens to ensure constant airflow. Alternatively, you can tie small bundles of mint tightly with twine and hang upside down in a cool and dark location for two weeks or use a dehydrator. The leaves are ready to be jarred when they are hard and brittle to the touch. Avoid light exposure during the drying process and dry at low temperatures of around 86°F.

Herbal Spotlight

During Victorian times, mint was referred to as "a treasure in the poor man's garden", referring to its multitude of uses yet inexpensive cost.

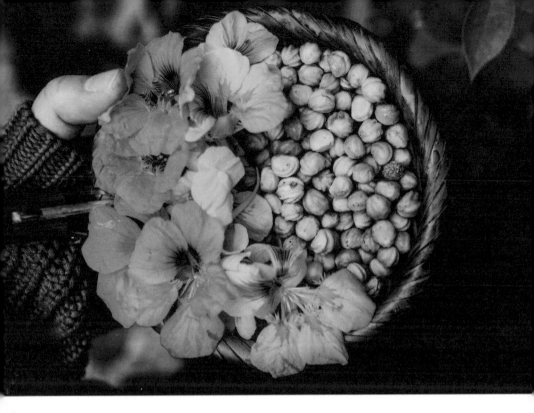

Nasturtium *Tropaeolum majus*

"Nasturtiums, who colored you, you wonderful, glowing things? You must have been fashioned out of summer sunsets."

—*Lucy Maud Montgomery*, writer (1874–1942)

Belonging to the Tropaeolaceae family, nasturtium is a vibrant and unique herb popular for its striking appearance and earthy, peppery flavor. It is most often used in culinary dishes, particularly salads and sandwiches. Its colorful blossoms and unique, lily pad-shaped leaves make it a popular ornamental addition to gardens. The trumpet-shaped flowers are usually vibrantly colored and come in a range of sunset colors. Nasturtium can be an annual or perennial, depending on the variety, and it can grow up to twelve inches tall. The plant is easy to grow and is often used in gardening as an attractive ground cover or climbing vine. I prefer to have it draping over the corners of my garden beds, mounds pillowing out of large containers, or cascading down hanging planters. All parts of the nasturtium plant are edible.

Beneficial Properties and Common Uses

Nasturtium has many beneficial attributes including antibacterial, anti-inflammatory, and immune-boosting properties that are used to naturally support those with sore throats, ear infections, colds, skin irritations such as eczema, acne, and psoriasis, and reduce swelling and inflammation. It is rich in vitamin C, iron, and antioxidants.

In the garden, it is a natural insect repellant and garden pest trap crop. It is also helpful in suppressing weeds in your garden beds and attracting pollinators, including bees and other beneficial insects. It grows well in containers and hanging baskets and is naturally deer-resistant. It is a good garden-bed companion to cabbage and radishes.

In the kitchen, I love to highlight the beautiful ornamental properties of nasturtium by using it fresh as a garnish or topping to add an elegant floral element and spicy kick to salads, pastas, charcuterie boards, and other savory dishes. The beautiful color of nasturtium is perfect for topping cakes, infusing in vinegar, or adding it dried and crumbled or blended into a powder to be mixed with salts and other seasonings. It can also be incorporated into herbal tea blends. Even the seeds are edible and can be pickled; it is sometimes called "the poor man's caper."

Try nasturtium in the recipes and tutorials on pages 192, 195, 221, 223, 242

To Grow

To grow, first soak your seeds overnight (approximately twelve hours) to soften the tough outer shell and expedite the germination process. Start seeds indoors four to six weeks before the last frost date for your zone. Plant the seeds one inch deep and cover completely.

Bottom-water, cover with a dome, and use a heat mat. Germination will take place in seven to ten days. Nasturtium does not tolerate cold temperatures, so I typically wait a couple weeks past my zone's last frost date before moving them from the greenhouse to the garden. Once in the garden, your seedlings will grow vigorously. If direct-sowing, wait until after the last frost date and when soil has warmed, and sow the seeds ten inches apart. It is not necessary to pinch nasturtium. Nasturtium is hardy in USDA zones 1–10.

Alternatively, starter plants are often available at your local garden center, and should be planted out after your zone's last frost date.

My favorite varieties of nasturtium are Ladybird Rose, Yeti, Orchid Cream, Cherry Rose Jewel, Tip Top Rose, Alaska Salmon, Salmon Baby, and Purple Emperor.

Care and Harvest

Nasturtium is a heat-loving plant that is easy to grow and thrives in bright, sunny growing spaces but can also tolerate partial shade. It prefers slightly acidic, well-drained soil. Provide a trellis for their vines to climb or space for their vines to cascade. If growing in the ground, give nasturtium ample space to stretch out and become a gorgeous groundcover of adorable lily pad leaves. Deadhead spent blooms regularly and prune back foliage occasionally to promote new growth. Nasturtium is considered a cut-and-come-again plant, meaning the more you harvest and prune, the more it will grow.

Harvest the flower heads just as they are beginning to open, using clean and sharp garden snips. If collecting entire vines to cascade down your vessel in a floral arrangement or to decorate a charcuterie board or garden table, check that the foliage has become firm and leathery.

At the end of the growing season, collect fallen seeds to dry and tuck away for next year, and then pull the plant and compost.

To Preserve

Nasturtium flowers and leaves can be dried by spreading them in a single layer on drying screens in a dark, cool location for about two weeks. They should be completely dry and brittle before crumbling, blending, or storing whole in an airtight glass jar. Alternatively, you can use a dehydrator. Nasturtium can also be pressed and used in botanical arts and crafts.

> **Herbal Spotlight**
> The name *nasturtium* is derived from the Latin word *nasus* meaning "nose" and *tortum* meaning "twister," most likely referring to people's reaction when smelling and tasting these peppery scented and flavored flowers.

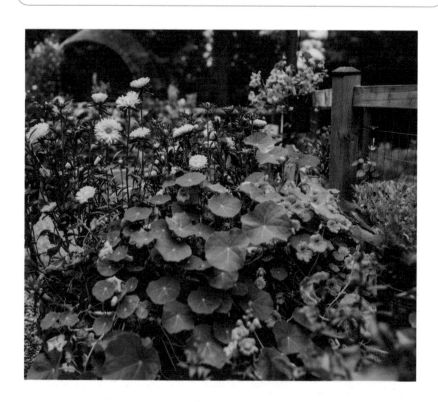

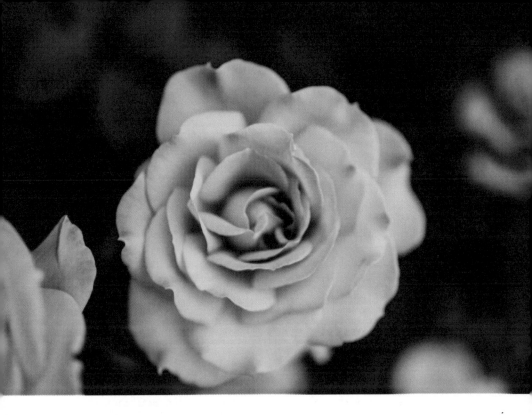

Rose *Rosa*

"It was June, and the world smelled of roses.
The sunshine was like powdered gold over the
grassy hillside."

—*Maud Hart Lovelace*, Betsy-Tacy and Tib (1892–1980)

Rose, a deciduous climbing or shrub-like perennial, has thorny stems and is known for its beautiful and fragrant flowers, which come in a variety of colors. The flowers are typically large and showy, with many petals arranged in a symmetrical pattern around a central cone-shaped structure called the receptacle. The leaves of a rose plant are typically green and oval-shaped, with serrated edges. The fruit of the rose, often referred to as the rose hip, also varies in color, shape, and size. They tend to be orange or red but may also appear as a deep purple or even black, and have a slightly sweet taste, with a delicious tang. Roses are a beautiful addition to any garden space. They are versatile and remarkably tolerant in many conditions, and have a long growing season. For the purpose of this book, I have included rose as an herb due to its extensive list of beneficial properties; however, it is worth nothing that rose is technically considered a shrub due to its combination of height and woody branched stems.

Beneficial Properties and Common Uses

The petals and hips of the rose have many beneficial properties. The petals are a rich source of vitamin C and antioxidants, and are used to naturally support those with anxiety, stress, digestive issues, and inflammation. Rose can be prepared a variety of ways, including as a cream, lotion, oil, ointment, tea, or tincture. Rose hips are rich in vitamins C, A, B1, B2, B3, and K, as well as flavonoids, tannins, and pectin, and are commonly used to naturally strengthen the circulatory system. Rose is considered a reproductive restorative in Chinese medicine, naturally aiding in infertility and hormonal imbalances, and regulating the menstrual cycle.

In the garden, rose attracts pollinators (particularly bees), repels many garden pests, and encourages an overall healthy garden ecosystem. Roses are an excellent garden companion to vegetables, and they have a long history of being grown together. They can even be used as a support system for vining vegetables such as runner beans and cucamelons. Roses are particularly good companion plants to marigold, lavender, catmint, allium, yarrow, and thyme.

In the kitchen, rose petals are edible and used most to flavor desserts, jams, teas, sugars, and baked goods. They are also beautiful as decoration atop cakes. Rose hips are also edible and can be used in powders, teas, jams, and syrups.

Around the home, roses are most commonly used in floral arrangements, bath soaks, scrubs, and salts, and dried roses are a beautiful addition to potpourri and floral arts and crafts.

Try rose in the recipes and tutorials on pages 195, 196, 198, 209, 215, 226, 231, 233, 235, 241, 249, 251, 262, 269, 270, 279, 285, 287

To Grow

Because growing roses from seed can be difficult and the plant will take several years to produce flowers, I recommend purchasing potted rose bushes from your favorite local nursery or bare roots from your favorite rose supplier. Choose a spot that receives a minimum of six hours of sun daily during the spring and summer months, with well-draining soil rich in organic matter. Break the soil up and supplement it with organic compost as necessary. Mix an organic rose fertilizer into the soil at this time, if desired. (This is an optional step.) Dig a hole that is deeper and wider than the container the rose came in, carefully remove the root base from the container, and gently break apart the roots or score them with a knife to encourage new growth. Place the root ball in the hole and backfill it with soil, tamping down as you go. Mound the excess soil slightly around the base of the plant, and then cover it with mulch. Finally, give your new bush a big drink of water. USDA zones 5–8 are ideal for growing roses. Some very hardy species of roses will grow in zone 4. If you live in zone 4, consult your local garden nursery for the types of roses that can withstand the cold and harsh weather conditions of your winters. Zones 9–11 can be too hot for some species of roses, so again, consult your local garden nursery for guidance on roses that may be able to withstand your high temperatures.

167

> "Roses do not bloom hurriedly; for beauty,
> like any masterpiece, takes time to blossom."
>
> —*Matshona Dhliwayo*, Canadian writer
> and philosopher

Considerations When Choosing Rose Varieties

Rather than list my favorite varieties of roses (there are far too many), I've decided it would be more beneficial to create a series of questions for you to consider prior to purchasing roses for your growing space, so that you can make an informed choice when investing in these beautiful plants.

- **Use.** Will your roses be strictly ornamental, or do you plan to harvest them for medicinal or self-care uses? Certain varieties of roses lend themselves to particular uses, so a bit of research can go a long way here.

- **Color.** What colors are you most drawn to, and what will coordinate with your existing perennials? This is important because some roses become very large and produce hundreds of blooms, so you want to really love the color you choose.

- **Characteristics.** What do you appreciate most about roses? Is it their fragrance? The size or quantity of the blossoms? The medicinal properties of their hips? Roses have many different fragrances, bloom sizes, designs, etc., so narrowing in on what is most important to you will be helpful in your shopping experience.

- **Location.** Where do you plan to plant it? Will it frame a doorway, stand erect along a border or pathway, or wrap up a trellis? Will it climb a wall or be planted in a larger container? There are varieties best grown in each of these living and growing situations.

- **Light.** What kind of sun does your growing space receive during the spring and summer months?

- **Pollinator-friendliness.** Does your variety attract beneficial insects who will benefit the rest of your garden?

Care and Harvest

Harvest rose petals on a dry morning when they are at their most fragrant. This should be done as soon as you see them beginning to bloom and before the petals are completely open. Rose hips can be harvested in fall when they have ripened and changed color. Rose hips are the fruit of the rose plant, which sets after the flower is pollinated in the early summer. The rose hips start out green and ripen to a bright orange, red, purple, or even black color in the fall. Simply snip just below the head of the hip to remove it from the plant. To process them, cut off both the blossom and stem ends and then slice the hip in half and scoop out the seeds in the center with the tip of a butter knife. The remaining flesh is the rose hip that should be used in recipes.

Roses need pruning to maintain an attractive shape and to keep them healthy. When pruning roses, take care not to remove the new growth shoots of summer varieties. These green, red, maroon, or purple shoots provide for next year's blossoms. Remember not to harvest or deadhead all your blossoms if you plan to harvest rose hips.

In the winter, cut back any foliage remaining from the fall. Remove any stems that show signs of damage, disease, or rot, and cut back the entire shrub to two-thirds its size. Always prune on an angle so that the tip of the clipped angle is on the outside of the plant and the shrub is rounded like a balloon.

To Preserve

There are several ways to dry rose petals. If you wish to keep the flower whole, simply harvest entire stems, tie them into a small bundle, and hang them upside down in a cool, dark place for two to three weeks. I prefer to harvest the individual petals from the plant without cutting the stem. This way, I leave behind the receptacle (center part of the rose) so that the hip can form, and I don't have to handle the thorny stems. Lay the petals in a single layer on drying screens for two weeks and then check back to ensure they are dry and brittle, or use a dehydrator. Rose petals can be steeped into simple syrups, frozen in ice cubes, infused into oils, or pressed and used in botanical crafting.

Herbal Spotlight
Nearly 200 percent of the recommended daily value of vitamin C is found in just an ounce of wild rose hips! So go ahead, give them a try!

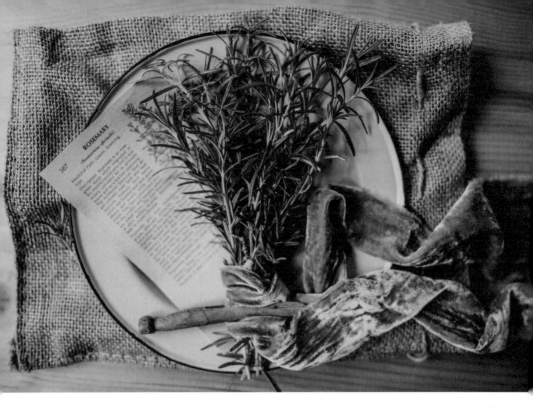

Rosemary *Rosmarinus officinalis*

> "There's rosemary, that's for remembrance;
> pray, love, remember..."

—William Shakespeare, Hamlet, Act IV (1564–1616)

A member of the Lamiaceae (mint) family, rosemary is a tender perennial shrub that can grow anywhere from two to six feet tall. It has dark greenish-blue, needle-like leathery leaves, and most varieties produce small pink, white, or blue flowers (though some varieties don't flower at all or only flower in warm climates). It has a distinctly lovely pine-like fragrance and a sweet but savory and slightly bitter flavor. It is sometimes called compass plant, compass weed, elf leaf, old man, herb of remembrance, sea dew, polar plant, Miss Jessopp's upright, dew of the sea, garden rosemary, or Mary's mantle.

Beneficial Properties and Common Uses

Rosemary has a long list of beneficial attributes, including antioxidant, antibacterial, antifungal antiseptic, diaphoretic, antidepressant, restorative, relaxing, uplifting, stimulating, and astringent properties that are used to naturally improve memory, enhance circulation, reduce fever, swelling, inflammation, and muscle tension, and soothe headaches, anxiety, exhaustion, and migraines. It is rich in vitamins A and C, and minerals including calcium, potassium, magnesium, phosphorus, iron, and zinc. It is commonly used to make essential oils, infused oils, teas, and tinctures.

In the garden, rosemary is naturally deer- and rabbit-resistant, repels garden pests, and attracts beneficial pollinators. Rosemary is a good garden-bed companion to brassicas (cabbage, broccoli, cauliflower, kale, brussels sprouts, rutabaga, turnips, etc.), beans, carrots, and sage.

In the kitchen, rosemary is used extensively in cooking, to season a variety of meat, poultry, fish, soups, and vegetable dishes, and infused in extra virgin olive oil to dip bread in. It also makes a beautiful garnish for dishes and cocktails.

Around the home, it is excellent as a floral arrangement filler and is commonly used in cosmetics and other skin-care products, perfumes, soaps, and shampoos.

Try rosemary in the recipes and tutorials on pages 192, 195, 198, 204, 209, 221, 226, 228, 231, 235, 242, 245, 262, 269, 270, 273, 275, 285, 287

To Grow

Because germination of rosemary seeds is generally quite low, I recommend purchasing rosemary starter plants from your favorite local nursery to plant out after your zone's last frost date. Rosemary prefers sandy, well-drained, and slightly acidic soil with a pH between 6.0

and 7.0. It also needs lots of sunshine, so choose a spot that receives a minimum of six hours of sun daily during the spring and summer months. Avoid planting rosemary in clay soil. Dig a hole that is deeper and wider than the container the rosemary plant came in, carefully remove the root base, and gently loosen the roots. Place the root ball in the hole and backfill it with soil, tamping down as you go. Mound the excess soil slightly around the base of the plant. Finally, give your new rosemary plant a big drink of water. Rosemary is most hardy in USDA zones 6–10.

If you decide to grow rosemary from seed, soak your seeds for twenty-four hours before sowing. Sow seeds ten to twelve weeks before your zone's last frost date. Surface-sow the seeds onto moistened soil and press down firmly but do not cover, as light is required for germination, which takes two to three weeks. Transplant outdoors after all threat of frost has passed. If you are growing rosemary as an annual, there is no need to space your rosemary more than eighteen inches apart. If you are growing rosemary in a warm climate as a perennial, give it twenty-four to thirty-six inches to grow to full size over several years.

Alternatively, starter plants are often available at your local garden center and should be planted out after your zone's last frost date.

Rosemary can also be grown from cuttings but can be a bit tricky. Learn more about the propagation method on page 93.

Care and Harvest

Rosemary needs very little care once it is established. Only water the plant when the soil feels dry, and harvest regularly or prune occasionally to keep the plant healthy. Harvest rosemary in the morning, after dew has evaporated off the leaves but before the sun is directly overhead. Snip sprigs off the plant with a clean pair of garden shears, leaving at least six inches of each stem behind so you don't deplete the plant's resources. Never cut the woody part of the stem, and only cut the top third of their length.

Rosemary does not overwinter well in cold regions. When temperatures reach 40 degrees Fahrenheit or lower, rosemary plants can be transplanted to a container with good drainage that is two times larger than the pot you purchased it in (or twice as large as its root system) and brought inside to a south-facing window until spring. Rosemary can be grown indoors or out, year-round. For indoor containers, create a soil mixture that is equal parts potting soil, compost, and sand. The Blue Boy variety is ideal for growing indoors.

To Preserve

Dry rosemary by tightly tying small bundles of rosemary stems and hanging them upside down in a cool and dark location. Check on it in two to three weeks by feeling the leaves. If they are stiff and no longer pliable, they are ready to be stored, whole on their stems, in an airtight glass container for up to a year. (You can remove the leaves from the stem if you wish, but be careful not to crush the leaves or it will release their flavor and potency.) Alternatively, a dehydrator can be used. Rosemary can be frozen in extra virgin olive oil or water.

173

Herbal Spotlight

In medieval times, some people believed that planting rosemary around your house could ward off witches and evil spirits. As a result, rosemary became known as the "herb of witches" and was often used in witchcraft and magic.

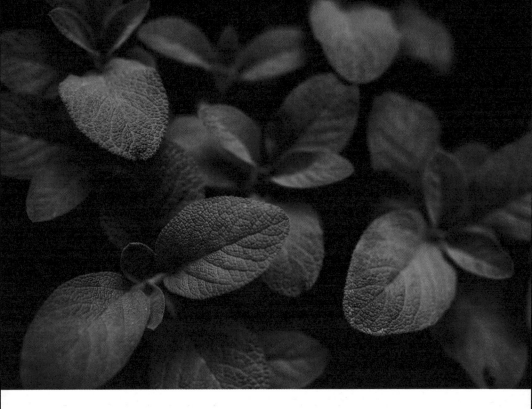

Sage *Salvia officinalis*

"Cur moriatur homo, cui salvia crescit in horto?"

—*Pliny the Elder*, Roman author, naturalist, and
philosopher (AD 23-79)

(old Latin proverb which translates to
"Why should a man die whilst sage grows in his garden?")

One of my favorite perennial herbs to grow, sage has beautiful grayish-green, light green, or sometimes purple leaves with soft velvety fuzz and bluish-purple flowers that thrive in a range of climates. With its versatile earthy, peppery flavor profile, it is used worldwide in many culinary dishes. It can be planted indoors or out and is easy to grow and maintain. It is sometimes referred to as common sage, traditional sage, wise sage, or garden sage. When planted outdoors, it attracts bees, butterflies, and other beneficial pollinators.

Beneficial Properties and Common Uses

Sage is another herb that is jampacked with beneficial attributes, including antioxidant, antimicrobial, anti-inflammatory, and cognition-enhancing properties that is naturally used to lower cholesterol, rebuild strength lost during an illness, elicit feelings of warmth and comfort, aid in menstruation and hot flashes, and relieve respiratory congestion. It is also used to relieve anxiety, blood clots, colds, depression, diarrhea, fever, gas, flu, migraines, and night sweats. Furthermore, it naturally supports those with Alzheimer's disease, dry skin, digestive issues, hair loss and graying, arthritis, and joint pain. It is rich in Beta-carotene, vitamins B1, B2, B3 and C, calcium, iron, and magnesium.

In the garden, sage is naturally deer resistant and is a good garden bed companion to rosemary, cabbage, and carrots. Do not plant near cucumbers.

In the kitchen, it is added fresh to a long list of savory dishes or can be used as a fresh or fried garnish, dried and added to spice blends and rubs, or infused as a tea. I also enjoy muddling sage in botanical cocktails, incorporating it into simple syrups, and garnishing dishes and drinks with it.

Around the home, it can be used as a natural mouthwash and its velvety foliage is an excellent floral arrangement filler. It also dries and presses well to be used in botanical arts and crafts.

Try sage in the recipes and tutorials on pages 192, 195, 198, 206, 221, 223, 226, 228, 235, 242, 245, 251, 261, 262, 269, 270, 273, 287

To Grow

Sage is an attractive perennial, and most varieties can be planted indoors or outdoors and live happily in the ground, in garden beds or in containers. It prefers loamy well-drained soil that has a neutral pH and full sun (at least six hours a day). Start seeds six to eight weeks

175

before your zone's last frost date by broadcast sowing them onto moistened soil and pressing them in firmly. Do not cover the seeds, as they need light to germinate (about three weeks.) Transplant outside after threat of frost has passed. If direct sowing, broadcast sow and cover the seeds very lightly with soil (no more than 1/8 inch) and keep the soil evenly moist for three weeks until germination. Thin out to 12 to 18 inches apart as they grow. It is hardy in USDA zones 4-10.

Alternatively, starter plants are often available at your local garden center and should be planted out after your zone's last frost date.

Sage can also be successfully grown from cuttings. Learn more about the propagation method on page 93.

My Favorite Varieties

While there are over five hundred varieties of sage, below is a short list of the ones I prefer to grow most:

- **Common sage (Salvia officinalis)**—most commonly grown in herb gardens for its flavorful and versatile profile, works well in many culinary dishes, particularly to spice poultry, stuffing, sausages, and vegetables; also called broadleaf sage or garden sage

- **Pineapple sage (Salvia elegans)**—bright and fruity but delicate scent and flavor like fresh-cut pineapple; leaves are a light green with brilliant red blooms in late summer; use both the leaves and the blooms to garnish desserts and mixed drinks; hummingbirds love it

- **White sage**—has a strong, pungent scent and has a rich history of ceremonial use by Native Americans tribes and is often used for smoke cleansing traditions to clear a space of negative energy; also called bee sage, sacred sage, or California sage

- **Greek sage (Salvia fruticose)**—smaller, more narrow leaves and a strong, pungent flavor commonly used in Mediterranean cuisine; pairs well with most meats

Care and Harvest

Water sage only when the soil around it is dry to the touch. Because it is a fairly drought-tolerant herb, it will most likely bounce back with a big drink of water even when it looks a bit wilted.

Harvest sage leaves regularly but always leave some leaves behind for the plant to use to regenerate. In late fall, do not prune the plant. Allow it to go dormant for the winter. Alternatively, you can make a temporary shelter for your sage plant using a piece of burlap and string.

To Preserve

Tightly tie a small bundle of stems together and hang upside down to dry or place individual leaves in a single layer on a drying screen. Alternatively, a dehydrator can be used. Preserve sage leaves whole in an airtight a glass container to preserve their flavor and potency.

177

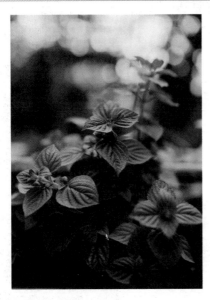

Herbal Spotlight
Did you know that smaller sage leaves are more potent and flavorful than the larger ones? Harvest smaller ones to use fresh and the larger ones for drying.

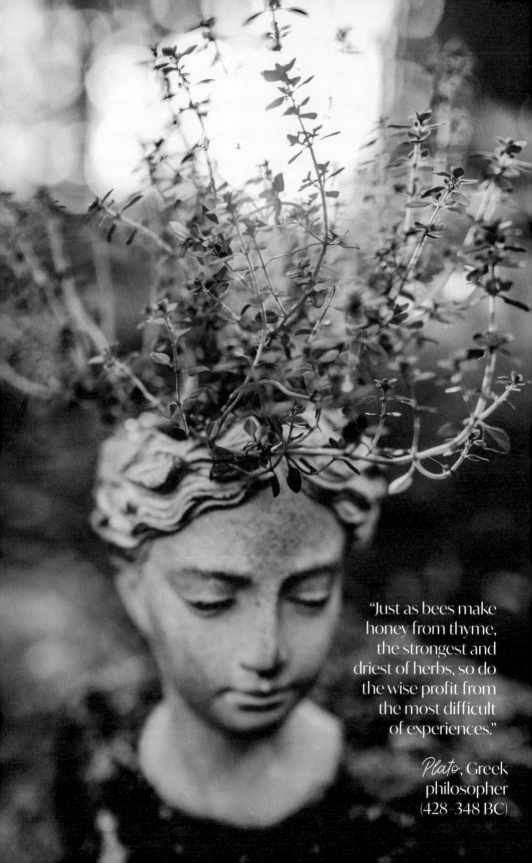

"Just as bees make honey from thyme, the strongest and driest of herbs, so do the wise profit from the most difficult of experiences."

—*Plato*, Greek philosopher (428–348 BC)

Thyme *Thymus vulgaris*

One of the most cherished herbs in my backyard garden, thyme is a fragrant evergreen perennial with small, delicate leaves that is often used to season and garnish a wide range of culinary dishes. Thyme leaves are typically green and have a slightly minty, earthy flavor with a subtle hint of sweetness. The herb is also known for its strong aroma, which is released when its leaves are crushed or rubbed. Thyme is a low-growing, shrub-like plant with woody stalks and fibrous roots. It grows anywhere from two to fifteen inches tall depending on the variety. Small, pretty flowers arrive during summer in dense, terminal clusters. The flowers can range from pale pink or magenta to white, blue, or lilac color. Other common names include garden thyme, common thyme, rubbed thyme, English wild thyme, German thyme, winter thyme, and the whooping cough herb.

Beneficial Properties and Common Uses

Thyme has many beneficial attributes, including antimicrobial, antifungal, stimulant, and expectorant properties that are used to naturally support respiratory issues, asthma, bronchitis, whooping cough, sore throat, infections, arthritis, digestive issues such as gas and heartburn, menstrual and uterine health, and circulation.

It is most used in the kitchen, is a popular ingredient in many cuisines and culinary dishes, and is excellent muddled into cocktails or garnishing botanical drinks and baked goods. Thyme also naturally preserves foods by preventing bacteria from growing on meat and keeping oils from going rancid.

In the garden, thyme attracts beneficial pollinators to your garden, including bees and butterflies, and is naturally deer- and rabbit-resistant.

Around the home, thyme is a popular ingredient in natural cleaning products and disinfectants.

Try thyme in the recipes and tutorials on pages 195, 198, 215, 221, 223, 226, 228, 235, 241, 242, 245, 262, 269, 270, 272

To Grow

Because thyme is very slow to germinate and has generally low germination rates, I recommend growing it from cuttings, using a method called propagation (see page 93) or purchasing starter plants from your favorite local garden center to plant out after all threat of frost has passed. Thyme thrives in sandy, rocky, dry, well-draining soil and full sun (eight hours a day) conditions. It will rot if planted in wet soil. Thyme is a natural garden pest repellant, so I recommend planting thyme throughout your garden along the perimeter of your garden beds. Thyme is hardy in USDA zones 4–9. In zones lower than 4, it can be treated as an annual.

To start thyme seeds indoors, sow your seeds six to eight weeks before your zone's final frost. Surface-sow onto moistened soil and press them firmly, but do not cover, as they need light to germinate. Germination will occur in approximately four weeks. Alternatively, you can direct-sow seed after all threat of frost has passed.

My favorite varieties of thyme are traditional, German, lemon, and lime.

> "I know a bank where the wild thyme blows, where oxlips and the nodding violet grows, quite over-canopied with luscious woodbine, with sweet musk-roses and with eglantine."
>
> —*William Shakespeare,* Midsummer Night's Dream (1564–1616)

Care and Harvest

Thyme needs very minimal care to be healthy. Thyme that has been planted in the ground can be watered regularly when soil near the base begins to feel dry. Thyme that is potted, however, should only be watered intermittently, letting the soil dry out between watering to protect it from root rot. Thyme will benefit from a dose of organic fertilizer every two weeks. If your plant begins to look exceptionally woody, you can cut some of the woody stems off completely (down to the ground) to encourage new, less woody growth. Never cut more than a third of your woody stems at one time.

To harvest thyme, cut the top four to six inches of the stems at any time during the summer months, preferably before blooming, with a clean pair of garden shears. I do not recommend harvesting from more than half of the plant at one time. Do not wash harvested thyme. Instead, shake it dry or rub it with a damp cloth to best preserve its volatile oils. Harvest flowers as they bloom to use fresh, or dry in the same way you dry the leaves.

To Preserve

Thyme is its most potent when used fresh, however, it can be successfully dried as well. To dry, hang sprigs upside down in a dark, dry area or place in a single layer on a drying screen for a week or more. Ensure the sprigs are brittle to the touch before storing them whole in an airtight glass container. When you are ready to use, remove the leaves from the stem, handling them carefully to retain their beneficial properties and aromatic oils.

Herbal Spotlight
Don't confuse common thyme (*Thymus vulgaris*) and creeping thyme (*Thymus serpullum*). While both have spreading growth habits, look quite similar, and are edible, common thyme grows more upright and is used for culinary and medicinal purposes, whereas creeping thyme hugs and grows along the ground (making its leaves dirtier) with leaves that are much smaller and quite tedious to harvest, so it is used primarily for landscaping.

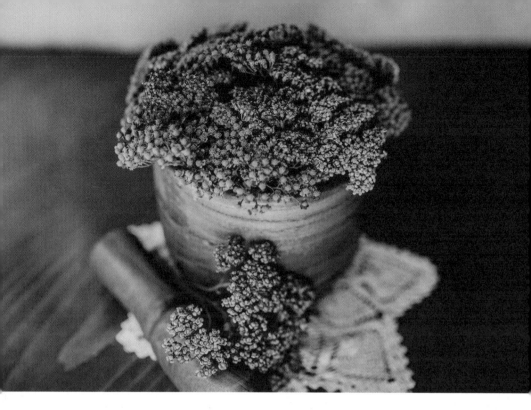

Yarrow *Achillea millefolium*

"Herbs, the gems of the plant kingdom,
have been prized for their medicinal properties
since time immemorial."

—*Mary Wilson Little,* American singer (1944–2021)

A member of the *Asteraceae* family, yarrow is a perennial that grows
two to three feet tall on a sturdy, erect stem with feathery leaves and
whimsical clustering flowers. I grow traditional white yarrow, as well as
pastel yellow and several shades of pink. Yarrow goes by many other
names around the world, including sweet yarrow, old man's mustard,
old man's pepper, field hops, devil's nettle, death flower, hundred-
leaved grass, woundwort, soldier's woundwort, arrow root, cloth of
gold, fern leaf yarrow, snake's grass, staunch weed, nosebleed, sweet
Nancy, carpenter's plant, and carpenter's weed.

Beneficial Properties and Common Uses

Yarrow has an impressive number of beneficial attributes, including antiviral, antiseptic, antimicrobial, and styptic properties that are used to naturally stop bleeding and regulate blood flow (which is where it gets the name "master of the blood") and aid in skin wounds, bee stings, colds, flus, fevers, upper respiratory congestion, menstrual cramping, and high blood pressure. It is rich in bioactive compounds such as alkaloids, camphor, terpenoids, and organic acids and is most commonly ingested as an herbal tea.

In the garden, yarrow attracts beneficial pollinators, including bees, butterflies, and other beneficial insects, and is a good companion to lavender, oregano, strawberries, brassicas, tomatoes, garlic, and onions. It is naturally deer- and rabbit-resistant. It has a deep root system, can tolerate drought conditions, and can help control soil erosion and improve soil fertility.

Around the home, I enjoy using yarrow for its gorgeous lacy texture addition to floral arrangements. It has an exceptionally long vase life.

Try yarrow in the recipes and tutorials on pages 209, 235, 262, 277, 279

To Grow

Yarrow is extremely easy to grow and thrives in dry, sandy, well-draining soil and in many different conditions. It prefers full sun, but will tolerate some shade or dappled light. It is considered both drought-tolerant and cold- and heat-tolerant. It grows happily in the ground, in garden beds, or in containers, but can be invasive, so I recommend growing it in a container. In fact, I typically broadcast-sow my seeds directly into containers in my greenhouse to save me from having to pot up or transplant. Avoid growing it in rich, moist soil, or it is likely to become leggy and flop over easily. To start indoors, sow seeds eight to ten weeks before your zone's last frost date, or sow directly into the garden two or more weeks after all threat of frost has passed.

Broadcast-sow over moistened soil and press firmly, but do not cover yarrow seed, as it needs light to germinate. Keep the soil moist using a mister or by bottom-watering until sprouts appear. Germination will take place in approximately two weeks. Harden off seedlings and plant outside after all threat of frost has passed. Yarrow can be found growing wild in meadows, grasslands, hedgerows, and woodland clearings, and is hardy in USDA zones 3–9.

Alternatively, starter plants are often available at your local garden center. I recommend planting out approximately two weeks after your zone's last frost date.

My favorite varieties of yarrow are Colorado Mix, Favorite Berries, The Pearl, and Cerise Queen.

Care and Harvest

Yarrow needs very little (if any) maintenance to grow. Deadheading spent flowers encourages new growth and blooming throughout the season. Water yarrow sparingly, but deeply when you do. On the hottest days, a drink of water will help revive a wilting plant. Yarrow has very aggressive underground rhizomes and will spread quickly, so keep this in mind when planting. If you already have an established yarrow plant, you can divide it (a process called root division) by carefully breaking the entire plant in half, separating the root system, and then transplanting the segments into different areas, which will each continue to multiply over time. I recommend dividing the plant every few years.

As with all other herbs, harvest yarrow in the morning, after the dew has dried from the plant but before the sun is directly overhead, to retain its beneficial oils and other properties. Harvest young yarrow leaves in the spring, preferably before the plant flowers. (Leaves sometimes reappear in the fall and can be harvested again at that time.) Harvest the flowers when the plant is in full bloom and their color shows vibrantly.

At the end of the growing season, cut your yarrow plant back to an inch above the ground. Be sure to label the location so you know where it will reappear next spring.

To Preserve

Yarrow is an excellent dried flower. To dry, bundle the stems tightly with twine and hang them upside down to dry in a cool, dark dry location for two weeks. Yarrow presses beautifully for use in botanical arts and crafts.

Herbal Spotlight
Native American tribes sometimes call the yarrow plant "chipmunk tail" due to the leaf's resemblance to the tails of the tiny creatures.

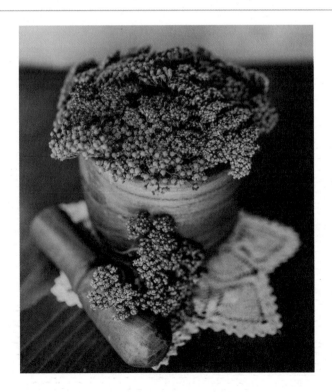

Part IV

Beyond the Garden

Seasonal Recipes, Tutorials, and Projects

The following pages contain a thoughtfully curated collection of recipes, tutorials, and projects that have been tried, tested, fine-tuned, and appreciated in my household. There are culinary recipes to explore how to add new flavors to your favorite dishes or new botanical notes to mixed drinks, crafting projects for those who like to create with their hands and work with botanicals, bringing the outdoors in, and self-care recipes to feel your best with the help of herbs from your garden.

Unless otherwise noted, all herbs used in the following four seasons of recipes are fresh and organic. When dried herbs are used or preferred, it is specified. All herbs used in simple syrups, infusions, self-care products, and culinary dishes and drinks should be organic and free of chemicals. Herbs given as gifts should also be organic and free of all chemicals.

When using essential oils, avoid contact with eyes, consult a doctor if pregnant or breastfeeding, and discontinue use if irritation occurs. If you are sensitive to a particular essential oil, always substitute or omit it from the recipe. When essential oils will have direct contact with your skin, it is important that they are properly diluted in a carrier oil. My favorite carrier oils are jojoba, sunflower seed, extra virgin olive, almond, avocado, and grape seed. Carrier oils should always be cold-pressed or virgin.

There are various supplies that would be good to have on hand, as they are needed for several of the recipes that follow. They are a double boiler, food processor (or coffee grinder), small saucepan, fine mesh strainer, grater, zester, organic cotton cheesecloth, natural parchment paper, twine, and clean, dry glass jars of various sizes with airtight lids. Spoons, spatulas, bowls of various sizes, measuring utensils, kitchen shears, scissors, cookie sheets, funnels with various-sized mouths, and wooden chopsticks or skewers will also be useful. Metal, wooden, or silicone molds are used in some recipes, but are often optional. Specialty supplies unique to a particular recipe or project have been listed in the ingredients list within the recipe. When foraging or trimming botanicals, garden snips and shears are recommended. Clear florist tape and 22-gauge green floral wire are also helpful for some projects.

Don't have a double boiler? No problem! To make a makeshift double boiler, use a glass measuring cup with a handle (Pyrex is my favorite brand for this purpose because they are sturdy and heavy) and place it inside a saucepan that contains two inches of boiling water. Be sure the handle of the glass measuring cup is hooked over the side of the pan so that it doesn't tip over if jostled by the boiling water.

187

To create many of the mixed drinks, refreshers, and cocktails, the following supplies will be helpful: ice cube trays and a supply of ice cubes, cocktail shaker, jigger, muddler, barspoon, and various fancy and fun glassware.

For recipes that call for beeswax, vegan wax alternatives include soy, carnauba, and candelilla.

Store balms, salves, lotion bars, butter, and infused and essential oils in a cool, dark location, such as a drawer, linen closet, or medicine cabinet. Avoid leaving in direct sunlight or extreme heat.

Spring

"It was one of those March days when the sun shines
hot and the wind blows cold;
when it is summer in the light,
and winter in the shade."

—*Charles Dickens* (1812–1870)

A Spring Awakening

The spring equinox, with its nearly perfect balance of day and night, is a reminder that longer, warmer days are ahead, bountiful harvests will be gathered, and new life will sprout. As the snow melts and the earth awakens from its winter sleep, an enchanting tapestry of fragrant herbs emerges. In this section, I've gathered my favorite recipes and tutorials made with those very first herbs to sprout during the waking days of spring, or with herbal oils that have spent the winter infusing in your pantry.

In the Kitchen

Chive Vinegars

One of the most kitchen-friendly herbs, chives are always among the first spikes of green to peek through the soil in my garden. It's such a treat to see them because it means longer, warmer days are just around the bend. With these recipes, you can choose if you'd like a bold or delicate base flavor of vinegar.

Bold Chive Vinegar Ingredients

1 cup (227 g) chives, chopped

2 cups (470 ml) white vinegar

¼ cup (57 g) lemon balm
leaves, torn or chopped

¼ cup (57 g) garlic, minced

¼ cup (57 g) shallots, chopped

Delicate Chive Blossom Vinegar Ingredients

2 cups (455 g) chive
blossoms, whole

2 cups (470 ml) white vinegar

To Create

1. Combine all ingredients in a clean, dry glass canning jar. Cut two small sheets of parchment paper and stack them on the mouth of the jar to prevent the vinegar from eroding the metal and then top with the lid, and twist to secure.

2. Give the jar a good shake and store at room temperature for two weeks, shaking daily.

3. Strain with a fine mesh strainer, coffee filter, or two layers of natural muslin cloth into a clean jar for storage.

Note: Have extra chives or chive blossoms left over? Add them to your cream cheese before whipping, or make chive blossom compound butter (recipe on page 192) or a finishing salt (recipe on page 270).

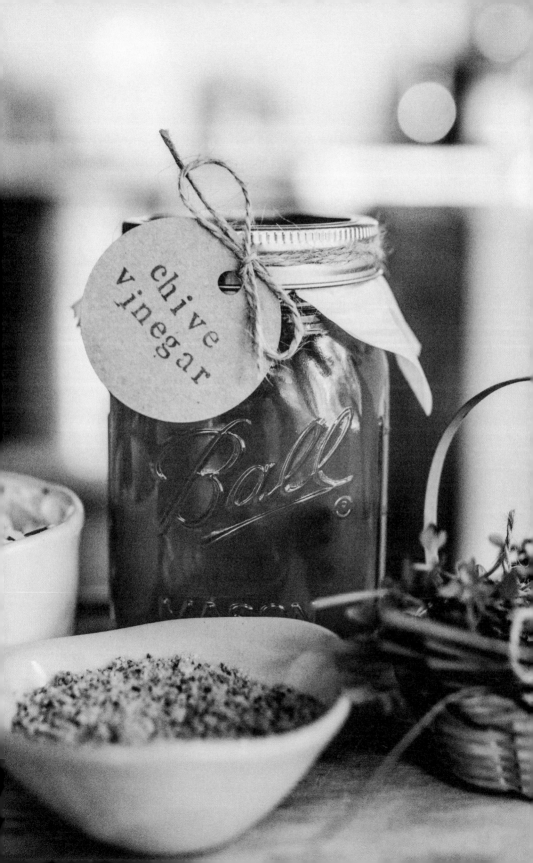

chive vinegar

Ball

MASON

Chive Blossom Compound Butter

One of my favorites, and a simple way to use fresh chives, is to make chive blossom compound butter. I grow common chives with delicate purple blossoms, but yours may be white, pink, or even crimson. Any variety can be used for this recipe. Compound butter can be used to add a delicate, buttery onion flavor and splash of color to fresh-baked bread, savory biscuits, morning eggs, mashed potatoes, or steamed vegetables, or be sprinkled on seafood or steak before serving. It can also be used as a base when making a roux or sautéing; it is a sweet and savory substitute for any recipe that calls for butter.

Compound Butter Ingredients

½ cup (115 g) butter, softened
2 tablespoons (30 ml) local honey
5 chive blossoms

5 tablespoons (71 g) chive, chopped
Himalayan sea salt to taste (start with ½ teaspoon [2 g])

Other savory herbs that would complement this recipe: 2 teaspoons (8 g) fresh chopped rosemary, 1 teaspoon (4 g) fresh chopped sage, 2 cloves fresh minced garlic, and/or 2 tablespoons (28 g) fresh nasturtium petals

To Create Compound Butter

1. Using kitchen shears, snip the chive leaves into small pieces until you have approximately five tablespoons (72 g).

2. Place your softened butter in a small bowl and add the chive leaves, blossoms, honey, and any other herbs you'd like to incorporate into the butter. Mix with your spatula until well combined.

3. Press the butter firmly into metal, wooden, or silicone molds, pushing in different directions to remove any air bubbles. Place in the freezer for fifteen minutes.

4. Carefully remove the butter from the molds (a firm tap against the counter may be needed) and store in a mason jar with small pieces of parchment paper between them. If you plan to gift

them with fresh bread, wrap them in brown parchment paper and secure with twine and a chive blossom. Alternatively, you can roll your compound butter into a log using parchment paper, twist the ends, and secure with twine or simply transfer the butter to a clean, dry canning jar with a lid.

Note: Compound butter made with fresh ingredients lasts a week in the refrigerator, especially if you add salt, or up to six months if wrapped tightly and frozen.

When harvesting chive blossoms, I recommend cutting the entire stalk near the base. While the blossom stalk is too tough to eat, it can be used as a handle while cleaning your delicate blossoms and then snipped off and composted.

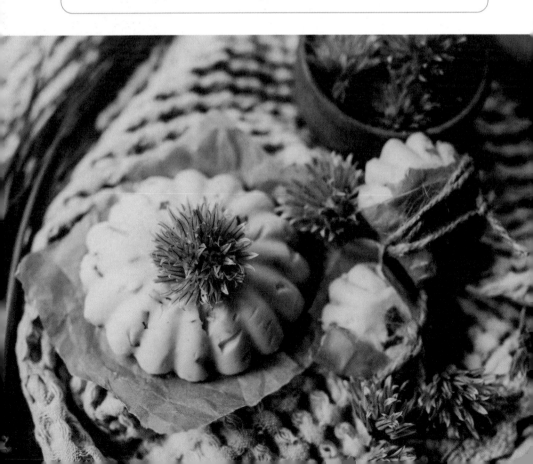

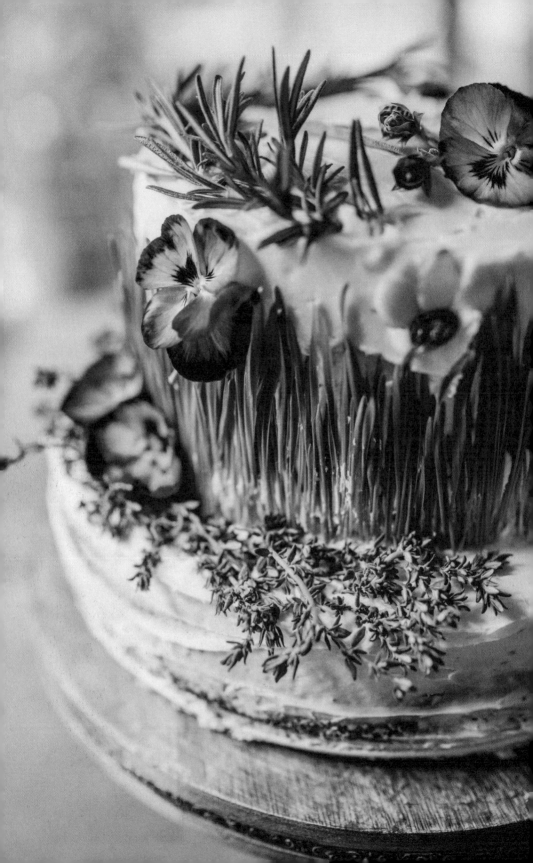

Culinary Decorating with Herbs

Decorating with fresh herbs from your garden is a simple and inexpensive way to make a big visual impact, adding color, texture, interest, flavor, and enchantment to baked goods. They can be added to cakes, cupcakes, or iced cookies after baking, using the frosting or icing to adhere them. Alternatively, they can be arranged atop cookie dough, pies, focaccia, breakfast pastries, or bread loaves *before* baking, letting the heat dry the herbs and meld them into the dough. Let the dough or a simple white icing be your blank canvas, using a combination of herbs to create a symphony of edible masterpieces.

Ingredients

baked good item(s) to
  be decorated

herbs of choice
frosting/icing if applicable

To Create

1. Bake your baked good item. Wait for it to completely cool or set, and then add your icing or frosting as you normally would.
2. Immediately after applying the icing or frosting, begin arranging the fresh herbs in place, pressing them gently into the icing, using the icing as an edible glue. Dab a bit of icing on the back of the plant pieces if necessary.
3. Refrigerate until ready to display or serve to prolong the herbs' freshness and prevent wilting.

195

Recommended Herbs for Decorating

- Bee balm
- Borage
- Chamomile
- Chive
- Fennel

- Lavender
- Lemon balm
- Lemon grass
- Lilac
- Mint

- Nasturtium
- Rose
- Rosemary
- Sage
- Thyme
- Viola

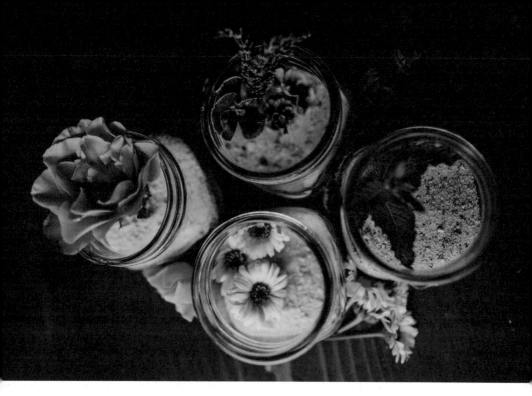

Botanical Sugars

This simple and beautiful botanical sugar recipe ignites all the senses, adding a hint of color, sweetness, fragrance, and herbal tones to your favorite drinks or baked goods in just minutes. In addition to using botanical sugars to coat the rims of drink glasses, try stirring a spoonful into hot and iced teas, or using it to make lemonade for a sweet and colorful twist. The sugars can add an herbal element to your favorite baked good recipe, sprinkled on your breakfast muffin, or mixed with jojoba or coconut oil to make a single batch of botanical sugar scrub. Botanical sugars also make beautiful gifts.

Ingredients

½ cup (115 g) herbs of choice

1 cup (227 g) white sugar for each type of herb

To Create

1. Combine sugar and a handful of the first selection of herbs in a food processor or coffee grinder. Process for thirty or so seconds until the herbs and sugar are well blended. Continue to add more herbs, a few pinches at a time, until you reach the vibrancy and strength of flavor and fragrance you desire.

2. Spread the botanical sugar onto a large clean plate or cookie sheet to dry out for one or two days, stirring a couple times a day. (A plate or pan with a lip will help keep the counter tidy.)

3. Once completely dry, store in a clean, dry glass jar with an airtight lid labeled with the herb and date created.

4. Continue these first three steps for each variety of herb, storing each botanical sugar in its own glass jar with label.

I recommend these herbs for their fragrant, colorful, and delicious properties:

basil—leaf green sugar
calendula—yellow sugar
lavender—vibrant purple sugar
lemon balm—vibrant green sugar
mint—light pale green sugar
rose—pink roses make a soft pink sugar
viola—purple violas make a gorgeous violet sugar

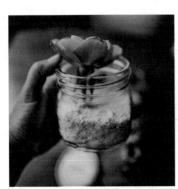

To use your botanical sugar to coat the rim of a drink glass, stir with a spoon to break up any larger pieces and pour a small mound onto a plate. Pour clean water into a bowl and dip the rim of the empty glass into the water and then into the sugar to coat it. Alternatively, dip one side of the rim into the water by angling the glass and then dip that same part of the glass into the sugar for an interesting look that gives the recipient the option to sweeten their sip, or not.

197

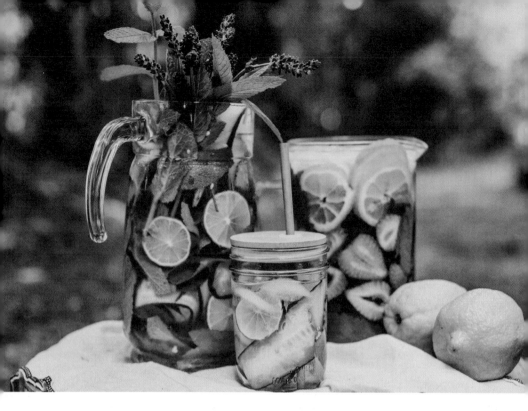

Seasonal Sips

Herbal Refreshers

Incorporating fresh-cut herbs from your garden is a simple yet delightful way to add a hint of natural flavor and aroma to your ice water beverages while incorporating revitalizing, detoxifying, and nourishing constituents and energetics that your body will appreciate. Experiment with different herb and citrus combinations to craft your own unique flavor profiles. If you'd like to sweeten your refresher, stir in a tablespoon or two (15–30 ml) of agave nectar or fresh local honey to each glass before serving.

Ingredients

large glass pitcher or jar
filtered water and ice
5 sprigs fresh herbs of choice

1–2 cups (227–455 g) fresh
   fruit, washed and sliced

To Create

1. Bruise the herbs slightly by clapping or rubbing them between your hands to express their essential oils.
2. If using fresh fruit, muddle a handful into the bottom of the pitcher or jar. Then fill your container three-quarters full with ice and water.
3. Add remaining fresh ingredients to a pitcher or jar of ice water, give it a quick stir, and serve. When time permits, a cold-infusion process can be implemented by letting your herbal water steep overnight in the refrigerator. The longer you steep, the more robust the flavors. The herbs from water that has steeped overnight may look a bit drab and need to be strained and replaced with fresh herbs before serving. Or, if you would like a clear herbal water, use a fine mesh strainer with a cheesecloth to strain all the fresh ingredient particles from the water. Serve over ice with an additional sprig of fresh herb for garnish.

Other herbs that would complement this recipe: basil, bee balm, borage, catmint, chamomile, lavender, lemon balm, lilac, mint (peppermint, spearmint, applemint, etc.), rose, rosemary, sage (common, honeymelon, pineapple, Scarlett tangerine), thyme (lime, lemonade, zesty orange)

Note: Your pitcher can be refilled with fresh filtered water multiple times over the course of your event or meal. Simply give your herbs a quick muddle and stir to release more of their volatile oils into the water before serving.

My Favorite Flavor Combinations

- Basil, Strawberry
- Bee Balm, Lemon
- Honeymelon or Pineapple Sage, Pineapple or Honeydew
- Lavender, Lemon Balm, Lemon
- Lemon Balm, Blueberry
- Mint, Cucumber, Lavender, Lime
- Mint, Strawberry, Lime
- Rosemary, Rose
- Sage, Honeydew
- Scarlett Tangerine Sage, Lemon
- Spearmint, Blackberry
- Thyme, Strawberry, Lime

Strawberry Fields Fizz

A spin on the Spring Fever created by Jamie Steinberg of Motel Morris in New York City, I first enjoyed this bright and bubbly drink on a warm spring evening in mid-June after returning from an annual strawberry-picking outing with my little ones. I've since enhanced the herbal notes in the drink by including mint simple syrup and substituting the elderflower syrup for elderflower liqueur. I substituted lemon juice for lime, bumping the refreshing notes up a notch and further complementing the sweetness from the strawberries.

Ingredients

4–6 ounces (120–177 ml)
  sparkling rosé wine, chilled
1 ounce (30 ml) elderflower
  liqueur, chilled

3 strawberries
½ ounce (15 ml) mint simple syrup
½ ounce (15 ml) lime juice
4 dashes bitters

Note: For an interesting twist, use chocolate mint to make the simple syrup and to garnish. It's like a chocolate covered strawberry in a cocktail!

To Create

1. Create the mint simple syrup according to the recipe on page 268.
2. Add the strawberries to a shaker and muddle.
3. Add the syrup, liqueur, juice, bitters, and some ice to the strawberries and shake until well-chilled.
4. Pour the entire contents into a wine glass and top with sparkling rosé. Give it a slow stir and garnish with a strawberry and borage blossom and/or mint leaf.

Note: To make this a nonalcoholic spritz, omit the bitters, wine, and liqueur, and add 3 ounces (90 ml) of sparkling juice and 3 ounces (90 ml) of elderflower-infused water or a nonalcoholic sparkling wine of choice.

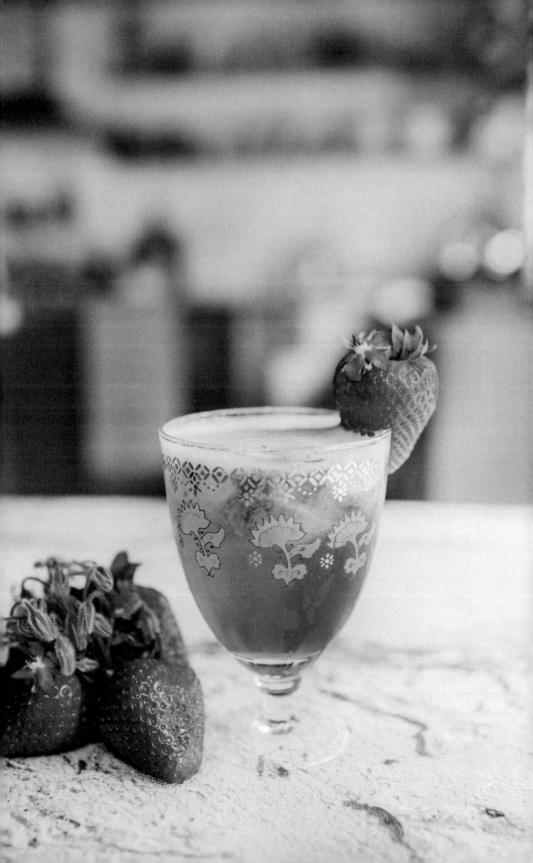

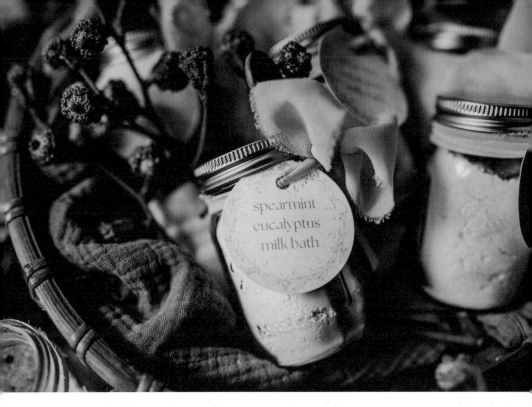

The Art of Self-Care

Spearmint Eucalyptus Goat Milk Bath Soak

This is one of my favorite self-care recipes and can be made in just minutes. I incorporate eucalyptus oil for its beneficial properties, including soothing dry, irritated skin, protecting against infection, and rejuvenating sore muscles. I chose spearmint oil to aid in reducing fever, fatigue, inflammation, and nasal congestion. Goat milk bath was chosen to moisturize and nourish skin.

Ingredients

1 cup (240 ml) dehydrated goat milk (available at organic groceries or specialty markets)

¼ cup (57 g) baking soda

¼ cup (57 g) cornstarch

10 drops eucalyptus essential oil

10 drops spearmint essential oil

pink Himalayan rock salt to finish

To Create

1. In a medium-sized bowl, whisk the first three ingredients until evenly combined.
2. Whisk the essential oils into the mixture to combine.
3. Funnel the mixture into a clean, dry glass jar and top with one tablespoon (15 ml) of pink Himalayan rock salt.

Precautionary note: Use caution when using this product, as essential oils can make certain bathtub surfaces slippery.

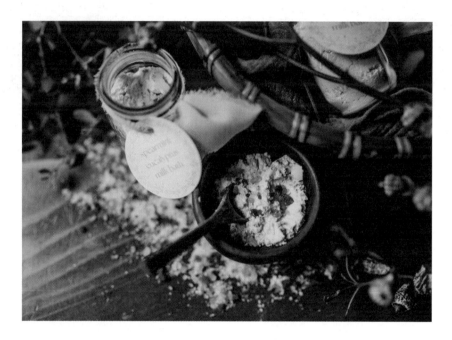

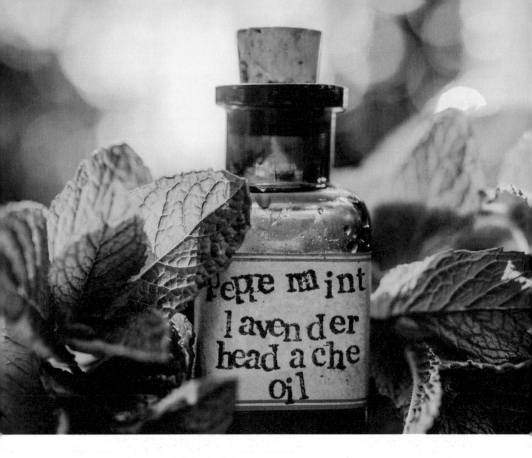

204 Lavender Peppermint Headache Oil

Headaches and migraines can be debilitating, and I've had my fair
share of them. Over the years, I've battled several types caused by
stress, tension, sinus congestion, and hormonal changes. This easy-to-
make oil is helpful to have on hand upon the onset of headache and
migraine symptoms. It can be stored in a small bottle with a cork or in
a capped roller-ball bottle, perfect for bedside tables and handbags.
When possible, after applying the headache oil, I find that taking a
big drink of cold water and then lying down in a dark, quiet room with
a cool, damp washcloth draped over my forehead is also a helpful
combination for decreasing the intensity of the ache or migraine.

Ingredients

25 drops peppermint essential oil
25 drops lavender essential oil
10 drops rosemary essential oil

3 teaspoon (15 ml) coconut
or sweet almond oil
(or blend of both)

To Create

1. Combine all the ingredients in a small bottle with screw top/cork/ dropper, or a roller-ball bottle with cap, cap or cork tightly, and shake well.
2. Store in a cool, dark place for up to eighteen months.

Precautionary Note: Always test out essential oil blends on a small patch of skin on your arm or leg before using on head, neck, or face. Always dilute essential oils as directed in this recipe before using on skin.

Suggested Treatments

◆ Migraine, stress, and hormonal headaches: massage on temples and back of neck

◆ Tension headache: massage on temples, back of neck, inside of wrists

◆ Sinus headache: message on temples, chest, and dab under nose

205

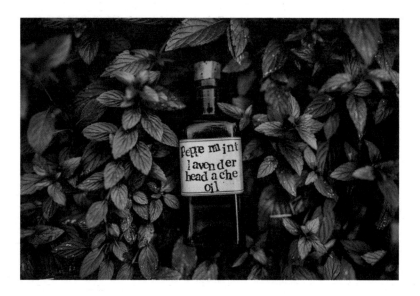

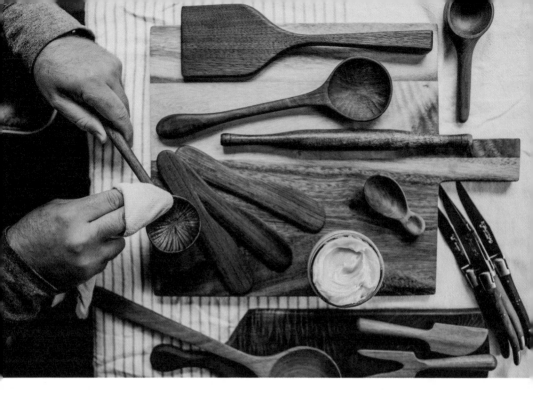

Garden-Made for the Home

Cedar House Woodenware Butter

Some of my most cherished kitchen items are handmade cutting boards and spoons my husband has made along with various wooden utensils and plates from amazing small shops. They encompass an old-world feeling in my kitchen that I appreciate. Woodenware butter nourishes the wood and enhances the natural colors, grain, spalting (wavey design), and chatoyancy (a metallic-like shimmer) present in the wood. Even if you hand-wash your woodenware, pieces can still begin to look drab over time, and a little care and attention will go a long way. This butter hydrates wood, restoring its vibrancy and grain details. I've also found that it softens wood, naturally repairing warping that occurs when your favorite pieces are accidentally run through the dishwasher or left outside in direct sun.

Ingredients

¼ cup (57 g) beeswax
¼ cup (60 ml) jojoba oil
½ cup (120 ml) juniper-
  infused oil blend

10 drops clary sage essential oil
  (or add dried clary sage when
  infusing your juniper oil blend)
15 drops lemon essential oil

To Create

1. Make infused oil blend according to the recipe on page 252.
2. Combine the first three ingredients in a double boiler over low heat and stir occasionally with a disposable wooden chopstick or skewer until completely melted and combined.
3. Remove from heat and stir in essential oils.
4. Carefully pour the mixture into a clean, dry, wide-mouth glass jar or tin and leave undisturbed to cool completely at room temperature.
5. Cap with an airtight lid and store in a dark, cool place like a kitchen pantry, cabinet, or the drawer for up to one year.

To use, apply a generous amount of butter onto wood with a cotton cloth dish rag or paper towel, rubbing the butter in small circular motions. Let the butter sit on the wood overnight, then wipe the excess butter off, and your boards and utensils are ready to use. In addition to kitchenware utensils, wood butter can be applied to butcherblock countertops and untreated indoor or outdoor wooden furniture.

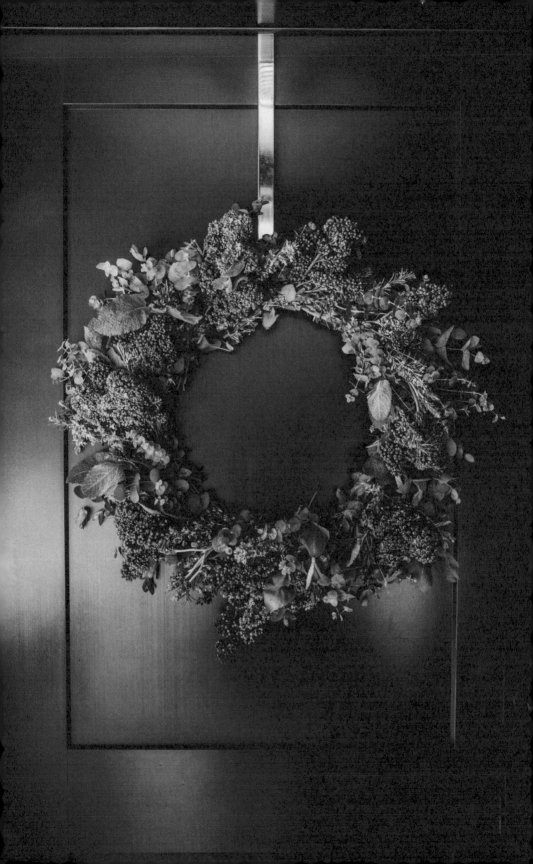

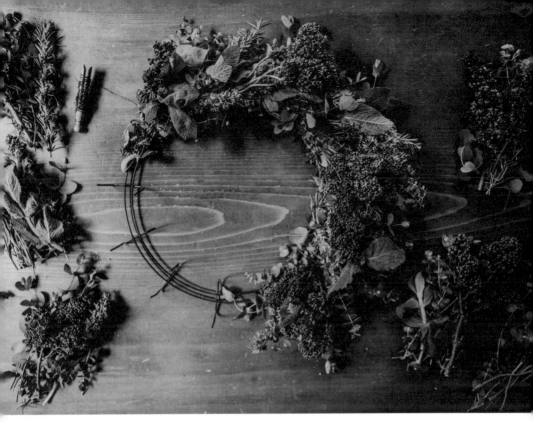

Tranquil Gardener's Wreath

The fragrant aroma of a fresh herbal wreath using herbs you grew
yourself is an herb gardener's delight. I most enjoy hanging mine
on our front door, in my kitchen above our stove to pluck from when
preparing meals and mixed drinks, or on our chicken coop door
to enjoy its fresh scent when I collect eggs. For this wreath, I used
a sixteen-inch (41-cm) wire wreath frame. Choose a wreath frame
appropriately sized for the area you plan to hang it. The wreath shown
is densely made and appropriately sized for a standard thirty-six-inch
(91-cm) door.

Ingredients

grapevine or metal wreath base
florist wire
12+ stems eucalyptus
  (1 gunni, 1 baby blue)
18 stems flowering rosemary

8 stems lilac

25 stems lavender

additional fragrant botanicals
of choice, fresh

> *Note:* Substitutions for eucalyptus could include fresh cedar, blue spruce, or juniper. I chose spearmint for its bright cooling scent and velvety texture, but any herb from the mint family would work well. I prefer English lavender because it is more fragrant than Spanish, flowering rosemary because the flowers complemented the other purple tones in the wreath, and lilac as the primary flower in season.

Other herbs that work well in wreaths: bee balm, calendula, chamomile, feverfew, marigold, rose, St. John's wort, yarrow

To Create

1. Attach the end of your florist wire to the base with a simple knot or by winding it around the outermost wire ring of the base a few times. Do not cut it. Leave it connected to the roll and continue to unroll as you secure the fresh materials.

2. Using a pair of garden snips or kitchen shears, create fifteen to twenty mini bundles of herbs, starting with eucalyptus as the base, and then clustering the other herbs on top as a second layer so they are all visible. No need to secure each bundle; small piles will do.

3. Fan out one of the botanical bundles and place it on the base, keeping the leaves pointed clockwise. Wrap the wire around the bottom of the bundle tightly three or four times where your thumb held them together. Do not cut the wire. Continue unwinding while wrapping and securing the bundles to the base in a spiral motion. (It's important to wind the wire around your bundles *very tightly*, as botanicals shrink as they dry.)

4. Attach the next bundle pointed in the same direction but just behind the first bundle, layering the herbs so that the "fan" of the second bundle covers the wire you used to attach the first bundle. Continue this step until the entire wreath is filled. The

number of bundles you need will vary, depending on how large your bundles are, how much you overlap each bundle, and the size of your wreath base.

5. When you are ready to attach the final herb bundle, tuck the base of the bundle underneath the fan of the very first bundle you secured. This will complete the circle and ensure all the florist wire is hidden. Then, give the wire a bit of a tail and cut it. Secure the end of the tail to the back of the wreath with a tight knot, creating a loop for hanging.

Note: To keep your wreath lush and green, hang outdoors where it is exposed to spring rainfall or mist it thoroughly with water every day. Alternatively, if you hang it indoors, you can choose to forgo misting and let the herbs dry on the wreath to be jarred together as a lovely herbal confetti blend to use in other recipes in this book.

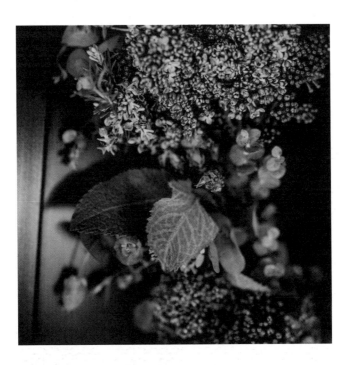

Summer

"It was June, and the world smelled of roses.
The sunshine was like powdered gold
over the grassy hillside."

—*Maud Hart Lovelace* (1892–1980)

A Shift to Summer

As we teeter between spring and summer, we begin to notice our gardens exploding with lush foliage and vibrant blooms. If it is true that the world speaks to us through the seasons, then nature is most definitely singing a botanical melody during these warmest months. Patiently anticipated since the first seeds were sown, we gather bountiful harvests to use in the following recipes until summer's final throes.

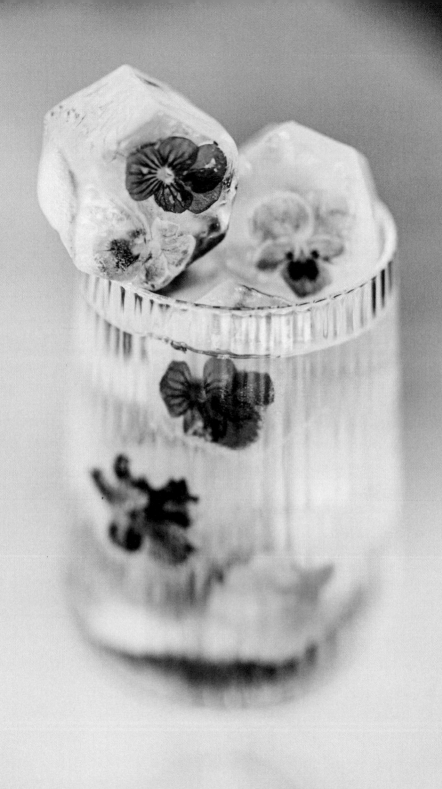

In the Kitchen

Herbal Ice Cubes

Send your guests swooning and elevate your iced drinks with these herbal ice cubes this summer. They are extremely simple to make and add whimsical flair to your favorite cocktails, mocktails, lemonades, spritzes, infused waters, and more.

Ingredients
fresh herb blossoms of choice
filtered water

Supplies
ice cube trays or silicone molds

To Create

1. Using a clean ice cube tray or silicone mold, fill it halfway with water. Place one or several botanical blossoms in each section. (I prefer a more simplistic look, so I typically only add one or two blossoms; however, cubes that are jam-packed with herbs can also be quite beautiful.)

2. Find a flat, level spot in the freezer for your ice cube tray to rest until frozen. If using a silicone mold, I recommend placing it on a plate and then placing the plate in the freezer.

3. Pull the tray from the freezer and fill it the rest of the way with water, then return to the fridge to freeze the top half of each cube. This two-part freezing process allows your blossoms to appear to be floating in the center of the cube, rather than on top.

215

Herb Blossoms Ideal for Ice Cubes

- borage
- calendula
- chamomile
- feverfew
- lavender
- lilac
- rose (petals)
- thyme
- viola

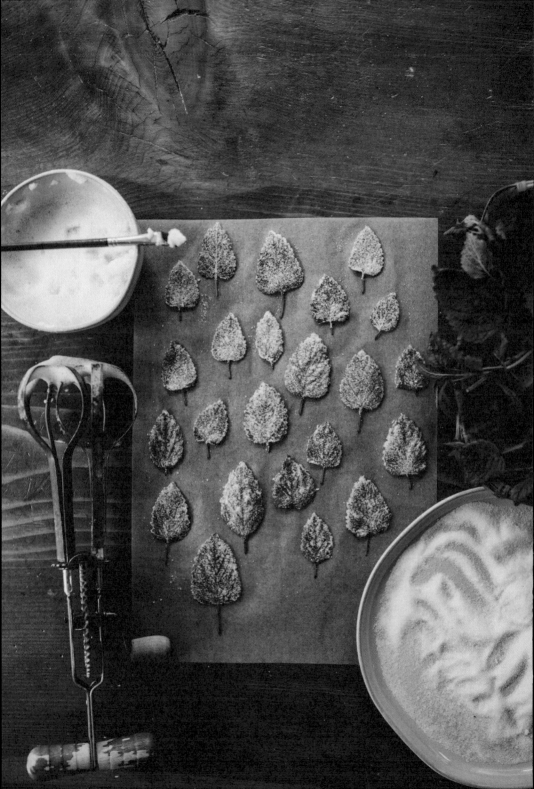

Candied Lemon Balm Cookies

Decorating baked goods with candied lemon balm is quite possibly my favorite use for this incredible herb, and the technique for making them is very simple, with supplies and ingredients you likely already have in your kitchen. They are the perfect addition to my traditional sugar cookie recipe, which I have altered just slightly to include a hint of lemon.

Ingredients for Candied Lemon Balm

bundle of lemon balm leaves

egg white from one egg

splash of water

½ cup (115 g) granulated sugar

To Create Candied Lemon Balm

1. Whip one egg white with a splash of water in a small bowl until very foamy.

2. Snip a single lemon balm leaf from your bundle, leaving an inch of the stem attached to act as a "handle" when brushing and coating the leaf. Using a soft-haired paintbrush, gently brush both sides of the leaf with egg white foam. If the egg white foam settles while you're working, rewhip it to keep it light and foamy.

3. Pour the sugar onto a small plate and lay the lemon balm leaf on top of the sugar. With a spoon, sprinkle sugar over the top of the leaf until fully coated. Then flip the leaf over and repeat on the other side. Gently relocate the leaf to a parchment paper-lined cookie sheet to dry overnight.

4. Repeat this process for as many leaves as you wish to make. Handle the leaves very gently, as they are fragile after they've been candied. I recommend making more leaves than the number of cookies you plan to bake, so you have extras to snack on or in case one breaks when being handled.

Ingredients for Cookies

1 cup (227 g) butter, softened
¾ cup (172 g) granulated sugar
1 egg

2 teaspoons (10 ml) lemon
 juice, freshly squeezed
2½ cups (570 g) flour

To Create Sugar Cookies

1. Mix the butter on medium speed in a stand mixer (or with a hand mixer) for thirty seconds. Add sugar, egg, and lemon juice to the butter and continue to mix until well blended.

2. Slow the mixer down to a lower speed and add the flour.

3. Remove from the mixer and knead for two minutes on a clean, lightly floured surface.

4. Store the dough in an airtight container or freezer bag and refrigerate overnight.

5. The next day, preheat oven to 375 degrees Fahrenheit and pull the dough from the refrigerator. Let it sit out on the counter until it is soft enough to be worked (but not room temperature), about thirty minutes.

6. On a floured surface, roll the dough out to ¼ inch thick and cut with a cookie cutter that is larger than your lemon balm leaves. Reroll the trimmings and continue until you've used all the dough.

7. Bake eight to ten minutes, until you see the bottom edges of the cookie very slightly beginning to brown. Transfer to wire racks to cool.

This recipe made ten cookies with a 2.5-inch diameter cookie cutter.

Ingredients for Glaze

2¼ cups (512 g) confectioner's
  sugar, sifted
2 tablespoons (30 ml)
  light corn syrup

2 tablespoons (30 ml) milk
1 teaspoon (5 ml) lemon
  juice, freshly squeezed

To Create Glaze

1. In a small bowl, mix all the ingredients with a fork until smooth.
2. Spread onto each cooled sugar cookie with a cheese knife. Snip the stem off a candied lemon balm leaf and center it on the wet glaze. Let dry for three or more hours before storing to be sure the glaze has dried completely.

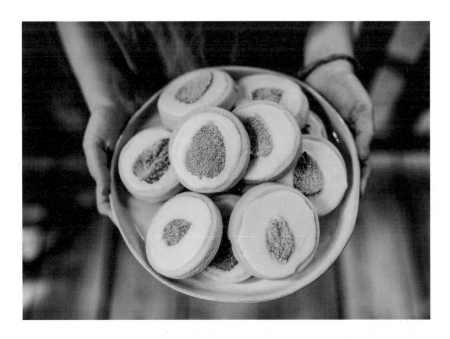

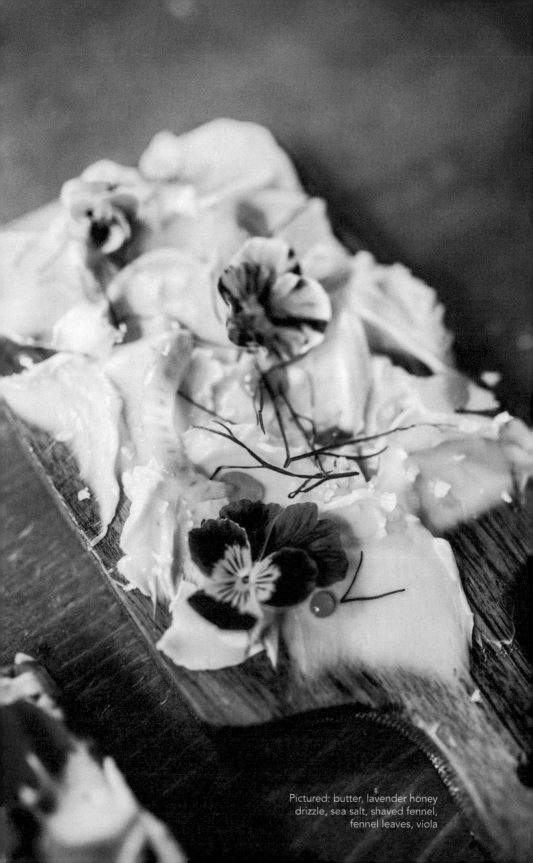

Pictured: butter, lavender honey
drizzle, sea salt, shaved fennel,
fennel leaves, viola

Sweet & Savory Butter Boards

A close cousin to the charcuterie board, the butter board is a new trend that's taken appetizers to a more refined level by prominently displaying fresh ingredients over a bed of smooth butter. My favorite board butter is Kerrygold Pure Irish Butter for its creamy texture, bold flavor, and rich gold color. It pays to splurge on a high-quality base for your boards. Also, don't limit yourself to butter as a base. Try spreading hummus, garlic paste or dip, goat cheese, or fruit dip on your board. Theme the flavor profile of your boards with sweet, spicy, savory, or a blend of these using your favorite combinations of herbs, spices, vegetables, fruit, seeds, and nuts. Below, I've created mini boards containing my four favorite ingredient combinations.

Ingredients

butter, softened to room temperature (or other base spread)

spicy honey (preferably locally sourced)

sea salt flakes

herbs of choice

other spices, vegetables, fruits, seeds and/or nuts of choice

To Create

1. Spread the softened butter evenly onto a clean, food-safe cutting or charcuterie board.
2. Drizzle honey over the butter, followed by a light sprinkle of sea salt.
3. Evenly sprinkle the fresh herbs and other ingredients over the butter, or get creative and use your fresh herbs to create a pretty "scene."
4. Serve with toasted bread, naan, biscuits, or crackers, and a few small butter spreaders to discourage double dipping.

Sweet ingredients: pomegranate seeds, honey, sliced fig, fig jam, sliced strawberry, sliced cooked pear or peach, sliced apple, dark or light raisins, dried cranberry or other dried fruit, brown sugar, lavender buds

Savory ingredients: arugula seedlings, microgreens, chive, viola heads, lilac blossoms, marigold petals, sage leaves, thyme, rosemary blossoms, shaved onion or fennel, fennel leaves, parsley, zinnia petals, nasturtium petals, basil, dill, pumpkin seeds, nuts (cashew, pine, pistachio, etc.), roasted garlic cloves, freshly shaved parmesan

Ingredients to add kick: crushed red pepper flakes, spicy honey, pepper jelly, mint leaves

Ingredients to add zest: lemon balm, bee balm, mandarin orange slices, lemon zest, olives, capers, sliced grapefruit

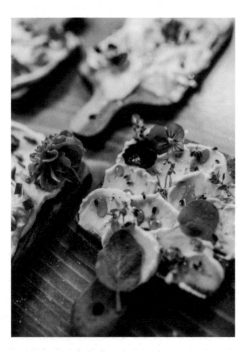

Pictured: butter, sea salt, spicy honey, sage petals, lemon thyme, lavender buds, viola

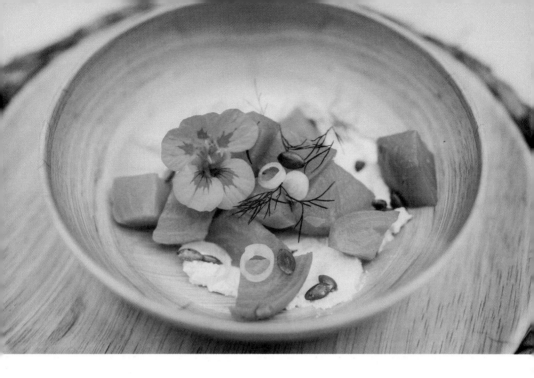

Summer Soiree Salad

This refreshing and vibrant beet and herb salad, served on a bed
of whipped honey goat cheese and drizzled with a nasturtium
vinaigrette, is packed with fresh seasonal ingredients. The robustness
of the nasturtium blossoms balances the delicate flavor of the fennel
perfectly, making it my go-to summer salad.

Vinaigrette Ingredients

½ cup (120 ml) extra virgin olive oil

3 tablespoons (45 ml) nasturtium
  vinaigrette (see recipe on page 242)

1 tablespoon (15 ml) Dijon mustard

1 tablespoon (15 ml) local honey

¼ teaspoon (1 g) salt

1 clove garlic, minced

To Create Dressing

1. Whisk all ingredients in a small bowl until completely combined.

   Note: Homemade vinaigrette will keep for seven to ten days
   when sealed with an airtight lid and refrigerated. If refrigerated,
   let it rest and come to room temperature after removing it from
   the refrigerator, and shake vigorously to liquefy any olive oil that
   solidified while it was chilled.

Salad Ingredients

10 ounces (255 g) log goat
  cheese, room temperature
2 tablespoons (30 ml) local honey
6–8 yellow beets
  (depending on size)
2 tablespoons (30 ml)
  extra virgin olive oil
a pinch or two of sea salt (to taste)

1 fennel bulb, shaved,
  fronds loosely chopped
salted pumpkin seeds
salt to taste
nasturtium blossom
1 cup (227 g) fresh
  arugula (optional)

Other herbs that complement this recipe: dill, mint, oregano, sage, thyme, bee balm, borage, calendula, chive

To Create Salad

1. Preheat oven to 375 degrees Fahrenheit.
2. Put the first two ingredients into a small bowl and whip with a hand mixer until smooth.
3. Wash your beets, scrubbing vigorously to remove all the dirt. Trim off the tops and bottoms and cut each beet in half.
4. In a bowl, toss your beet halves in olive oil to coat.
5. Create a large foil "boat" on a baking sheet by molding a large piece of tinfoil into a cup-like shape with a large flat bottom. Place your beets on the tinfoil boat, creating a single layer. Add 3 tablespoons (45 ml) of water to the bottom of your tinfoil boat, close and fold the top of foil, and roast for one hour.
6. Pierce the largest beet with a fork to check that it is cooked to your liking. The fork should be able to easily puncture through to the middle of the beet.
7. Let the beets cool to room temperature, then, using a paper towel, gently press and wipe the outside of each beet to remove the skin. The skin will easily slide off.
8. Cut the beets into one-inch cubes and put back into the bowl you used to coat them with oil. Add the vinaigrette and toss again to evenly coat the beets.

9. To assemble, lay out your small serving-sized plates and spread a smear (approximately 2 ounces [57 g]) of whipped goat cheese on each. Divide the beets evenly over each goat cheese smear, sprinkle with salted pumpkin seeds, shaved fennel, fresh fennel leaves, and a pinch or two of sea salt, and garnish with a fresh nasturtium blossom.

    Note: If you would prefer a more traditional salad, add ½ heaping cup (115–125 g) of fresh arugula on top of the whipped goat cheese for the beets to lie on.

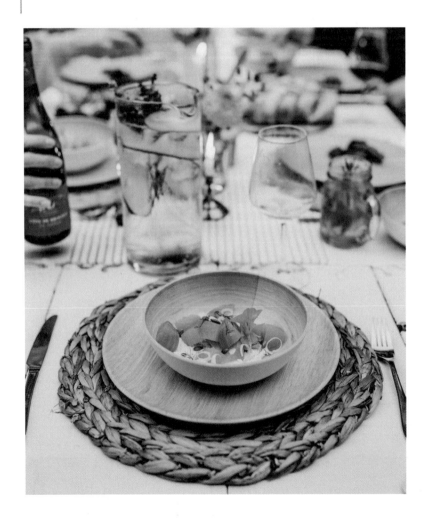

Seasonal Sips

Lavender Lemon Balm Lemonade

This herbal twist on everyone's favorite summer refreshment is sure to hit the spot on those hot summer days and is an excellent way to bring fresh lavender and lemon balm from garden to table.

Ingredients

1–2 cups (227–455 g) lemon balm, plus a few additional leaves to garnish

6 cups (1,440 ml) filtered water

3–4 cups (950–1,190 ml) lemon juice, freshly squeezed

1 cup (240 ml) lavender simple syrup

5–10 English lavender stems

1 lemon, sliced into wheels

To Create

1. Make lavender simple syrup according to the recipe on page 268.

2. While the simple syrup is cooling to room temperature, muddle the fresh lemon balm into the water and set aside to infuse for at least an hour in the fridge, or overnight, if possible. Strain the lemon balm from the water and pour into a glass pitcher before moving on to the next step.

3. Add the juice and syrup to the pitcher and stir.

4. Add ice and lavender stems to the pitcher and serve over ice, garnished with one of the lavender sprigs, a lemon wheel, and a lemon balm leaf.

Note: As alternatives to lemon balm-infused water, substitute the lavender simple syrup for the Beez Kneez simple syrup recipe on page 269, or infused honey with lavender and lemon balm as shown on page 241.

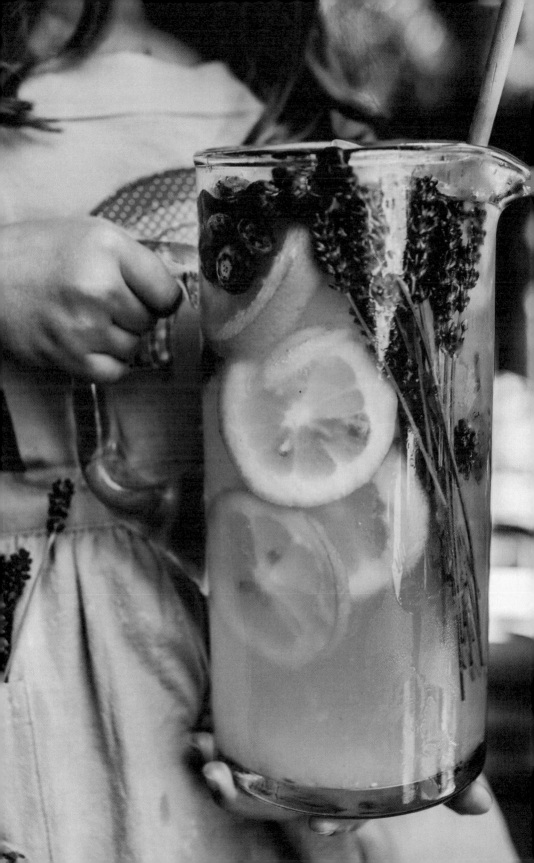

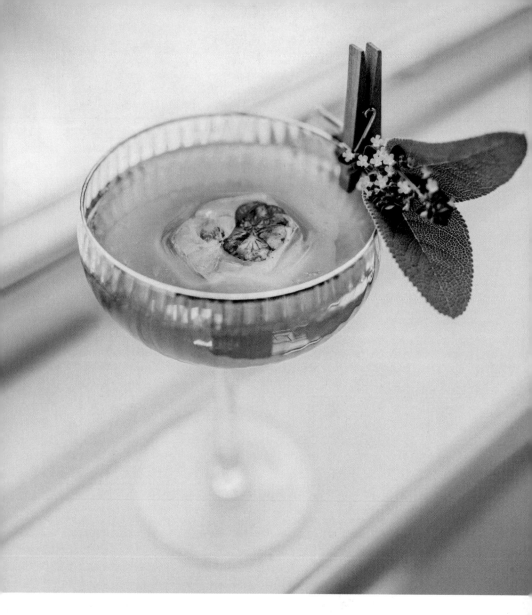

Garden Goddess Cocktail

Subtle floral notes from the Crème de Violette complement the herbal earthiness from the freshly muddled herbs and simple syrup in this handcrafted botanical cocktail. And now that your garden is stocked with fresh herbs, you can easily manipulate the notes in this drink to fit your personal taste.

Ingredients

2 ounces (60 ml) pineapple-
  infused vodka
½ ounce (15 ml) Crème de Violette
½ ounce (15 ml) Earth
  Song simple syrup
1 ounce (30 ml) lime juice,
  freshly squeezed

6 dashes bitters
1–2 ounces (30–60 ml) cold water
1 sprig rosemary
3 sage leaves (common
  or Scarlett tangerine)
1 sprig thyme and 1 sage
  leaf for garnish

Note: The variety of sage you choose to muddle will alter the drink's herbal notes. I prefer to use common broadleaf sage to add earthiness, which balances the sweetness from the pineapple-infused vodka. Using Scarlett tangerine sage will add distinct floral notes. I've found that the flavors of fruit-themed varieties of sage, such as pineapple or honeymelon, get lost in the pineapple-infused vodka, but are a great option if you are forgoing the fruit-infused spirit step.

To Create

1. Make the Earth Song simple syrup according to the recipe on page 269.

2. Make pineapple-infused vodka by filling a large glass mason jar with cubes of fresh or canned pineapple. Pour vodka over the pineapple until it is completely submerged, approximately 8 oz (240 ml) of vodka for every ½ cup of fresh pineapple. Give it a good shake and store in a cool, dark place for five days, shaking occasionally. Strain the fruit from the vodka.

3. Combine first seven ingredients in a shaker with a half-cup of ice and shake vigorously for fifteen seconds.

4. Strain into a coupe glass.

5. Garnish with a thyme sprig and sage leaf.

Note: To make this cocktail a mocktail, substitute the vodka with one ounce of pineapple juice and one ounce of water.

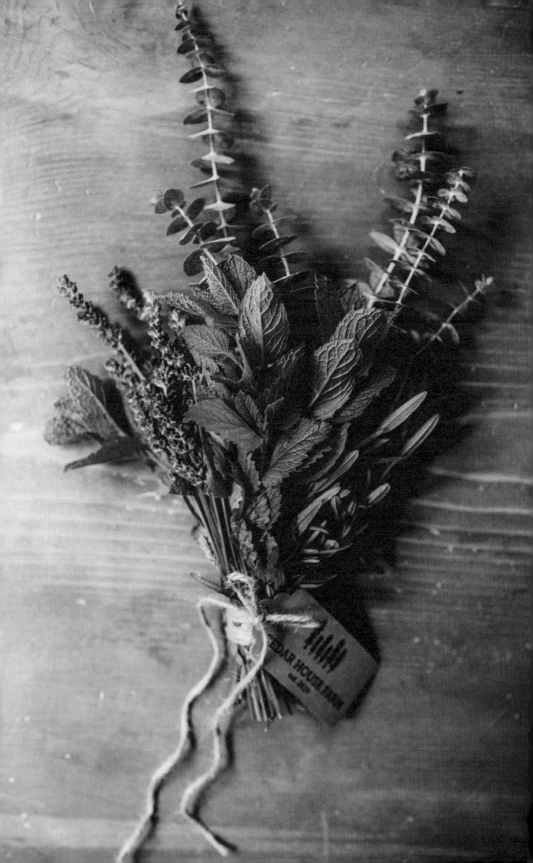

The Art of Self-Care

Aromatherapy Herbal Shower Bundle

This mood-lifting herbal shower bundle is a beautiful fragrant addition to any bathroom. They provide a rejuvenating aromatherapy experience each time you bathe or shower, improve the air quality of your bathroom space, and absorb extra moisture in the air. When tied upside down around the neck of your shower head, the steam from your shower releases beneficial aromatherapy oils into the air while hydrating the herbs, extending the life of the bundle. Alternatively, the bundle can be treated like a bouquet and placed in a vase of water on a windowsill, shower shelf, or sink counter, for the same effect. When gifting, include a gift tag or note to share directions for use along with the benefits of each herb with the recipient.

Ingredients

5 stems eucalyptus

10 stems lavender

5 stems lemon balm

5 stems mint

5 stems rosemary

> *Note:* Any combination of the ingredients that are readily available to you can be used for this project. Peppermint and spearmint are most widely used from the mint family and will be easiest to source in large bundles for this project.

> *Note:* Eucalyptus holds water in its stems and will easily outlast all the other herbs in the bundle. Lemon balm, on the other hand, is often the first herb to wilt and needs to be plucked from the bundle.

Other herbs appropriate for this recipe: bee balm, chamomile, rose, lilac, juniper

Aromatherapy Benefits

Eucalyptus—refreshing, clarifying fragrance that aids in respiratory ailments

Lavender—fresh, tranquil, relaxing aroma with calming effect

Lemon Balm—bright, uplifting aroma helps soothe anxiety, nervous tension, insomnia, and headaches

Mint—invigorating, refreshing scent provides respiratory support to ease congestion

Rosemary—fresh, pungent fragrance enhances circulation and brain function, and eases headaches and migraines

To Create

1. Gather your botanical ingredients. Remove any broken or blemished leaves. Rinse and shake dry.

2. Create a bouquet starting with the longest-stemmed plants, bunching them together at the base. Layer with shorter herbs, fanning them out slightly as you go. Continue to layer until you've used all the herbs.

3. Secure with twine, wrapping tightly. Tie a double knot and/or bow, leaving eight inches or so of length on each of the ends of string for tying to the shower head.

4. Cut the ends of the stems to an even length for a clean finished look.

Add a Seasonal Touch

Spring—3–5 stems lilac

Summer—3–5 stems fresh cottage roses or small bundle of chamomile

Autumn—2 cinnamon sticks or dried apple slices

Winter—2 dried citrus slices and red velvet ribbon

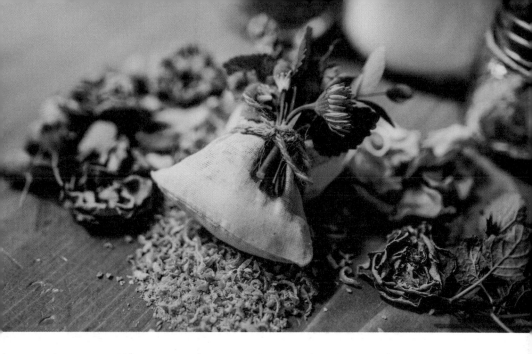

The Gardener's Bath Tea

I wanted to bottle the calming energy of my backyard garden into a bath soak that would cleanse the mind and ease tired muscles and joints after a day in the garden. I chose each of these herbs for their detoxifying, stress-relieving, and soothing properties. I added the lemon peel for its antioxidant properties, and the salts were chosen to help soothe aching muscles and give your skin a boost after prolonged sun exposure. Muslin bags are a great no-mess alternative to dropping the bath soak mixture directly into your bath water and can be tied to the faucet while drawing your bath. Then, let the bag float in your bath for continued aromatherapy. You've nurtured your garden all year. Through this bath soak, your garden will return the favor.

Ingredients

2 cups (455 g) Epsom salt

1 cup (227 g) Himalayan
 pink rock salt

1 cup (227 g) lavender buds, dried

1 cup (227 g) lemon balm, dried

1 cup (227 g) rose petals, dried

1 cup (227 g) calendula, dried

1 cup (227 g) eucalyptus, dried

1 cup (227 g) chamomile, dried

1 cup (227 g) dried lemon
 peel shavings, dried

10 drops eucalyptus essential oil

10 drops lavender essential oil

10 drops lemon essential oil

2 tablespoons (30 ml) sunflower oil

reusable muslin tea bags

Note: This recipe makes six to ten soaks, depending on the size of the tea bag. To make a single-use soak, reduce the Epsom salt ingredient from 2 cups to 2 teaspoons, remaining dry ingredients from 1 cup to 1 teaspoon, and then add one drop of each of the essential oils and four drops of sunflower oil. If making a single-use soak to use the same day, fresh herbs and lemon peel can replace dried.

Other herbs that would complement this recipe: bee balm, mint

To Create

1. Dry the lemon peel by grating the peel of a clean organic lemon and leaving it out on a drying screen or parchment paper-lined cookie sheet for a few days until dry. Alternatively, to speed up this process, place the cookie sheet in an oven on the lowest setting (150 degrees F is ideal) for ten minutes at a time until dry, or use a dehydrator.

2. In a large bowl, combine the salts, dried herbs, and dried lemon peel.

3. In a separate small cup, combine the oils and drizzle them into the mixture, stirring thoroughly.

4. Scoop into muslin bags and tie the drawstring tightly.

Precautionary note: Please use caution when using this product, as the oils can make certain bathtub surfaces slippery.

Note: Sunflower oil is used as the carrier oil in this recipe to fit the garden theme; however, any cold-pressed or virgin oil can be substituted. Coconut, sweet almond, grapeseed, and olive are good alternatives. Carrier oils are necessary to dilute essential oils that will touch your skin.

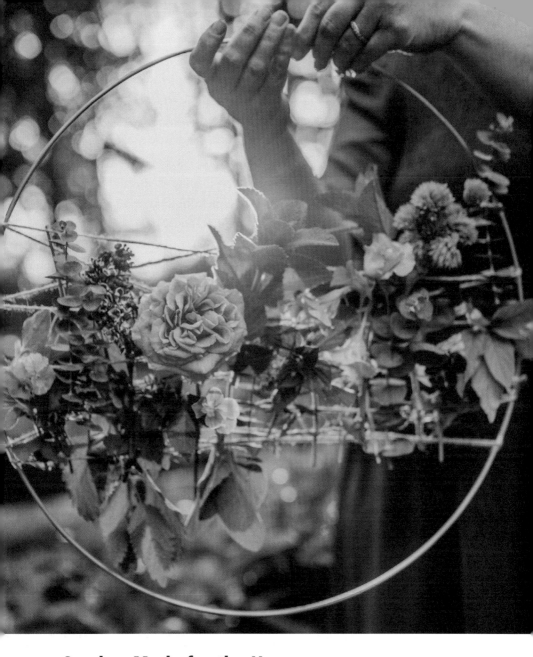

Garden-Made for the Home

Tied and Tucked Herb Drying Hoop

There are some activities that simply feed the soul. For me, this craft is one of them. It inspires time in the garden harvesting herb clippings, considering which colors coordinate well and which herbal blends will be most useful to have on hand in small quantities. Then begins the slow, peaceful process of working with your hands to create with the herbs you've been caring for all these months. The end result is an ephemeral piece of botanical art with a cottage garden essence that embodies scenes from the season. It can be displayed in your home to dry (I hang mine above my stove so I can pick from them to use when I'm cooking), then the herbs can be dismantled and jarred.

Ingredients

herb clippings of choice   metal floral hoop

Herbs that work well for this project: bee balm, calendula, chamomile, chive blossoms, echinacea, eucalyptus, juniper, lavender, lemon balm, lilac, marigold, mint, rose, rosemary, sage, thyme, yarrow

To Create

1. Cut a piece of twine to roughly ten times the diameter of the hoop you're using. Tie one end to the hoop with a simple double knot.

2. Pull the twine across and through the hoop and wrap it around the opposite side. Use a small piece of clear tape to keep it from sliding. Continue weaving the twine back and forth in a figure eight motion with irregular angles, securing the twine to each side of the hoop as you go. Space the twine and crisscross it so it intersects in different places. When you reach the end of the twine, tie it tightly to the hoop with another double knot.

3. Vertically weave the herb clippings through the twine and reposition the aerial parts to your liking. Be creative with how you incorporate the herbs. You could hang them upside down or upright, staggered or linear, spaced out or closer together. Hang your finished hoop where you can enjoy simplistic botanical beauty while they dry.

Note: I used an eighteen-inch hoop in this sample. As an alternative to metal floral hoops, embroidery hoops can be used and come in a variety of sizes.

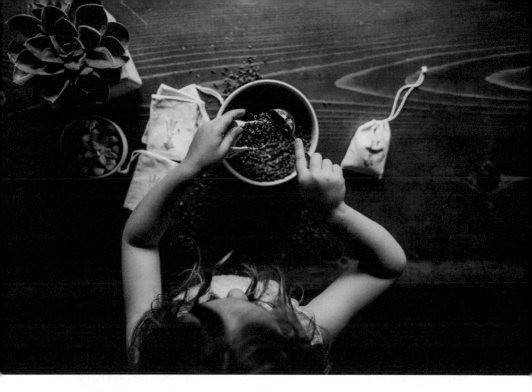

Lavender Sachets

Lavender sachets are a simple and useful late summer craft to use any
remaining lavender bundles at the end of the season. To easily remove
the dried buds from their brittle stems, gather a handful of stems and
roll them between your palms over a large bowl or basin. The buds will
fall right off, leaving just the stems to be composted.

Ingredients

4 cups (910 g) dried lavender buds

8 drops lavender essential
  oil (optional)

8 3.9-x-3.15-inch natural cotton
  muslin drawstring bags

To Create

1. Place the lavender buds in a bowl and stir in the essential oil.
2. Personalize the muslin bags with a lavender, logo, or event-
    themed stamp, if desired.
3. Spoon approximately ½ cup (115 g) of buds into each muslin bag
    and tie the drawstrings tightly into a tiny bow.

Note: If you are short on lavender, you can substitute half of the lavender with dry rice and increase the lavender essential oil drops from eight to twelve.

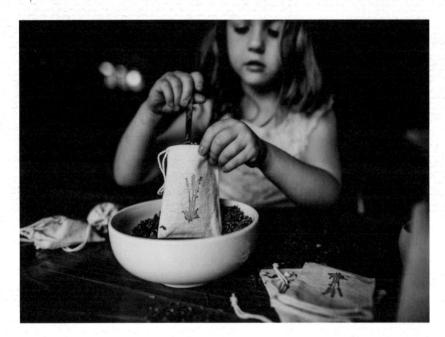

Autumn

"And all at once, summer collapsed into fall."

—*Oscar Wilde* (1854–1900)

Autumn Shows Herself

And just like that, summer dwindles to autumn. Even though it happens every year without fail, it always surprises me how quickly the summer months soar by. Beginning in October, fog rolls onto our property, streaming through the trees, spotlighted by the morning sun. It's one of my favorite parts of autumn on our homestead, and it reminds me how much I've come to rely on the rhythms of each season. How much they balance us. With the help of the autumnal equinox, we gravitate toward the comfort and warmth of our home during this season. May these projects and recipes inspire you to use those final harvests from your herb garden and to begin experimenting with the herbs you've dried this season.

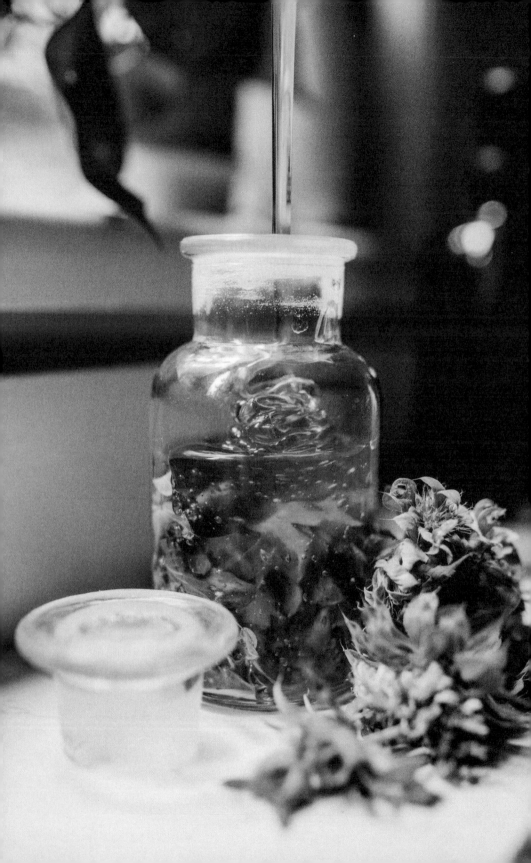

In the Kitchen

Bee Balm Honey

One advantage of living in the woods is having neighbors who keep bees. I grow bee balm and other herbs that feed our neighboring bees, and then my neighbors process the honey, which ends up gifted back to us, an agricultural ecosystem at its core. This fragrant and flavorful recipe is so easy and versatile, you'll wonder why you haven't done it before now! The honey can be used in both hot and iced teas and lattes, on fresh sourdough bread or biscuits, or by the spoonful to help soothe cold and flu symptoms.

Ingredients

bee balm, dried (amount will vary depending on size of storage container)

honey, preferably locally sourced (amount will vary depending on size of storage container)

To Create

1. Add a bit of honey to the bottom of a clean, dry glass jar—just enough to coat the bottom. Fill the jar three-quarters full with the bee balm, but do not pack tightly.
2. Pour honey over the bee balm. Use a chopstick or skewer to move the blossoms around, to make sure they are completely saturated and that there are no air bubbles.
3. Cap with an airtight lid and let sit for a week before removing the plant parts.

> *Note:* You can substitute dried bee balm for fresh; however, the moisture from fresh herbs will expedite the crystallization process of honey. If using fresh bee balm, refrigerate the infused honey to delay crystallization and extend shelf life. If using dried bee balm per this recipe, your honey can be kept out on your counter for up to six months. Store your honey in glass containers, as it will erode plastic.

Other herbs that work well with this recipe: anise hyssop, calendula, chamomile, lavender, lemon balm, lemon thyme, lilac, and rose.

Nasturtium Vinegar

Nasturtium, with its vibrant flowers and large round lily pad-like leaves, is not only gorgeous cascading down your garden containers, but the flowers, leaves, stems and even seeds are all edible! Nasturtium blossoms are a beautiful garnish for salads, dinner plates, and pretty much any savory appetizer dish or charcuterie board. Use them to create a finishing salt, infuse vodka to give your Moscow mules a kick, or, as shown here, create a beautifully bright nasturtium vinegar to use as a base for salad dressings.

Ingredients

vinegar, white wine, or
  distilled vinegar
1 heaping cup (227 g)
  nasturtium blossoms

1 sprig rosemary
1 large handful chive, chopped
1 small handful
  whole peppercorns

Other herbs that would complement this recipe: sage, thyme, oregano

To Create

1. Add all the ingredients to a large glass jar. Before securing the lid, cut two small sheets of parchment paper and stack them on the mouth of the jar to prevent the vinegar from eroding the metal. Shake well.
2. Store in a cool, dark place for two weeks, shaking daily.
3. Strain and bottle to separate the plant material from the infused vinegar. The nasturtium turns the vinegar a gorgeous vibrant orange color, making it an impressive gift.

To make a simple vinaigrette, add three parts extra virgin olive oil for every part vinegar, add a pinch each of salt and pepper, shake vigorously, and serve.

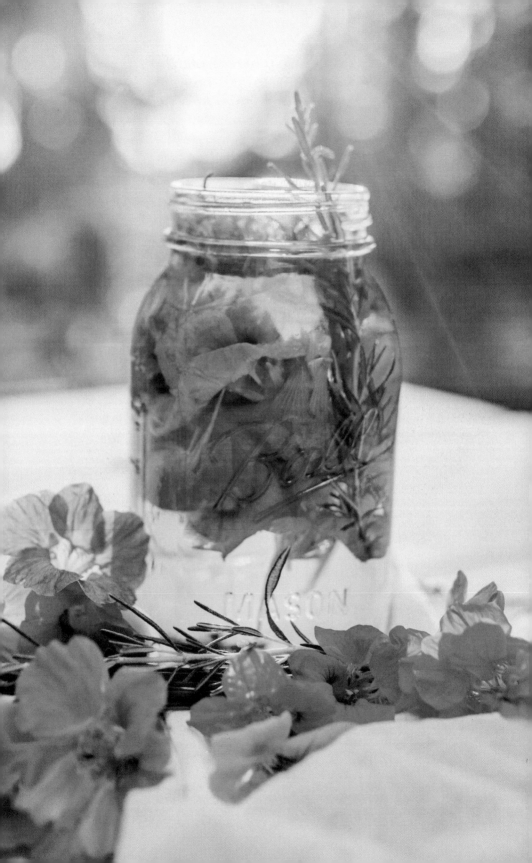

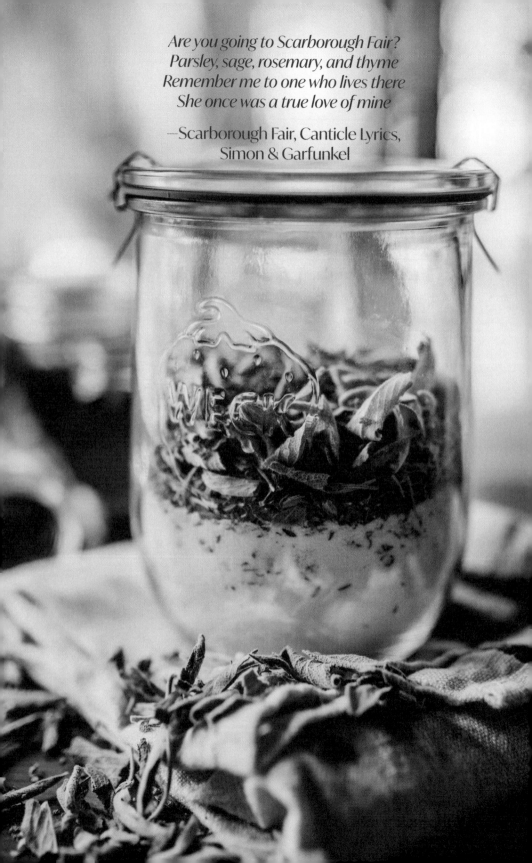

Are you going to Scarborough Fair?
Parsley, sage, rosemary, and thyme
Remember me to one who lives there
She once was a true love of mine

—Scarborough Fair, Canticle Lyrics,
Simon & Garfunkel

Scarborough Turkey Brine

Brining a turkey is a culinary technique that involves soaking the bird in a solution of sugar, salt, water, and often other flavor-enhancing ingredients. This process not only adds moisture to the turkey but also infuses it with savory herbal flavors, resulting in a tender and succulent centerpiece for your holiday feast. The salt in the brine helps to break down the proteins in the meat, allowing it to retain more moisture during cooking for an extra juicy bird. If you've never brined your turkey, it's a game changer and guaranteed make for a memorable holiday feast.

Ingredients

1 cup (227 g) sea salt

1 cup (227 g) sugar

2 tablespoons (28 g)
 parsley, dried

3 tablespoons (42 g) sage, dried

3 tablespoons (42 g)
 rosemary, dried

3 tablespoons (42 g) thyme, dried

To Create

1. Combine all ingredients in a clean, dry glass jar and secure with an airtight lid. Shake well.
2. Store in a cool, dark place until the morning before you want to roast your turkey.

To Use the Brine

1. Unpackage your turkey, remove the giblets, and transfer it to a stockpot. The stock pot you choose should be large and deep enough to hold your turkey entirely submerged in water. If you can't find one large enough, a food-safe bucket is an alternative.
2. Next, make space for the pot in your refrigerator and test to make sure it fits with the lid on before moving on to the next step. I find this to be the trickiest part of the entire process! (If it won't fit with the lid, use plastic wrap to cover.)
3. Heat 1 quart of water just enough to warm it to the touch (about a minute in the microwave). Stir in the brine mixture until

completely dissolved and pour over the turkey. Add additional water by the quart until the entire turkey is submerged. Cover and place in the refrigerator for twenty-four hours.

4. When you're ready to roast, remove your turkey from the solution, rinse, and pat dry so you still get that crispy delicious skin everyone fights over! Dress and roast as you normally would.

Note: Brined turkeys sometimes cook more quickly than those not brined, so check the internal temperature of your turkey an hour or two earlier than you normally would.

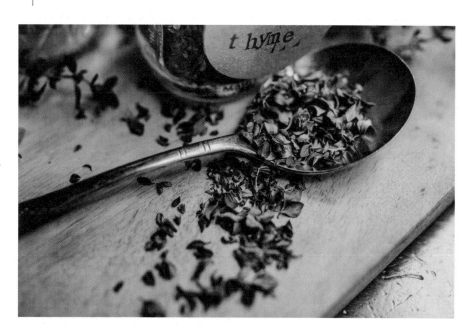

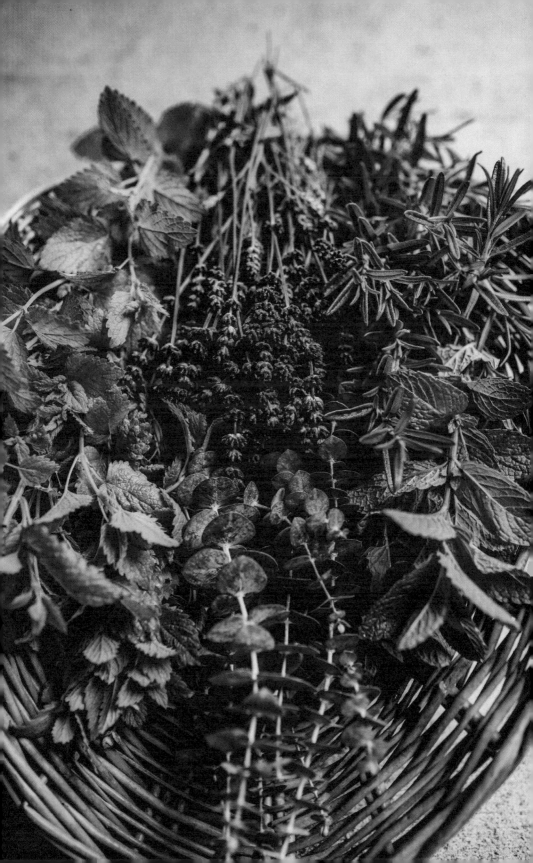

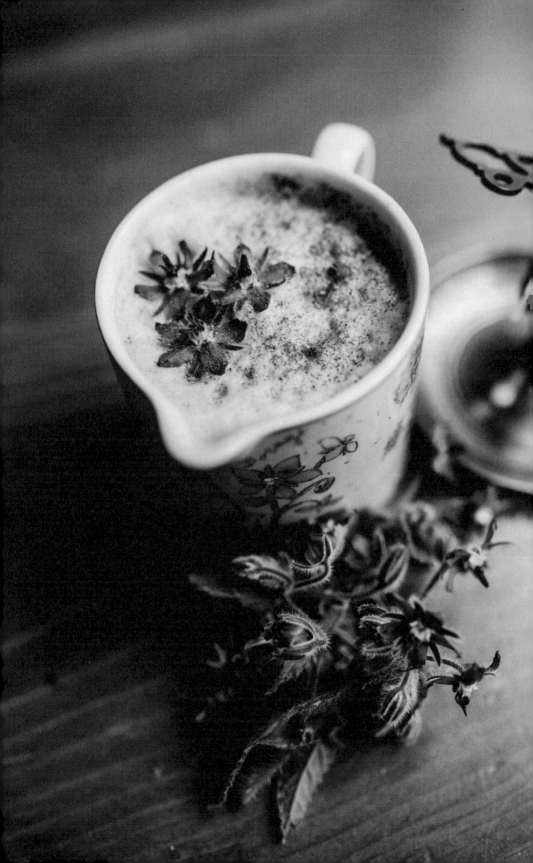

Seasonal Sips

Floral Fusion Latte

Borage, with its subtle yet sweet taste, pairs perfectly with lavender and rose to create a simple syrup base that is perfectly floral in this breezy botanical coffee drink. Enjoy hot, as the recipe suggests, or over ice on a summer day by omitting the frothing process and pouring the ingredients over ice.

Ingredients

2 shots espresso

1 tablespoon (15 ml) Floral
  Fusion simple syrup

8 ounces (240 ml) milk, frothed

ground cinnamon

borage blossoms to garnish

To Create

1. Make Floral Fusion simple syrup according to the recipe on page 269.

2. Extract two shots of espresso from your espresso machine, Nespresso machine, French press, or moka pot.

3. Stir the simple syrup into the espresso until well combined in the bottom of your favorite mug.

4. Froth your preferred milk (I use whole or 2 percent for best froth) and pour over the espresso mixture, stirring lightly.

5. Top with lots of foam, a pinch of ground cinnamon, fresh borage blossoms, and/or a sprig of lavender.

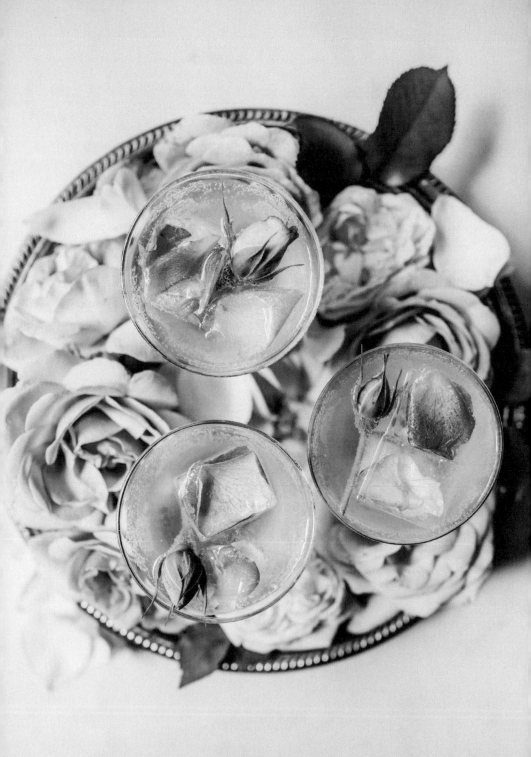

Blush Rose Gimlet

As rose season bows to a close, put the last of your roses to good use in this delicately flavored gin gimlet. This enchanting cocktail combines the timeless elegance of a classic gin gimlet with the subtle floral notes of rose petals and elderflower, creating a sensory experience that is both refreshing and captivating. The crisp and botanical essence of gin harmonizes seamlessly with the citrusy tang of fresh lemon juice and orange bitters, while the delicacy of the rose simple syrup and rose petal ice cubes imparts a subtle and aromatic layer of sophistication. Each sip unfolds like a stroll through a blooming garden.

Ingredients

2 ounces (60 ml) gin

1 ounce (30 ml) elderflower
  liqueur, chilled

¼ ounce (7.5 ml) lemon juice

½ ounce (15 ml) rose simple syrup

5 dashes orange bitters

champagne or Prosecco,
  a generous splash

rose petal ice cubes

fresh rose bud or sage leaf

To Create

1. Make rose simple syrup according to the recipe on page 269.
2. Make rose petal ice cubes according to the recipe on page 215.
3. Combine the first five ingredients in a shaker with ice and shake vigorously for fifteen seconds until well-chilled.
4. Strain over rose petal ice cubes into a coupe glass.
5. Garnish with a fresh rose bud, blossom, petal, or sage leaf.

> Note: To make this cocktail a mocktail, substitute the gin and liqueur with lemon or elderflower-infused water, soda water, or a nonalcoholic spirit of choice.

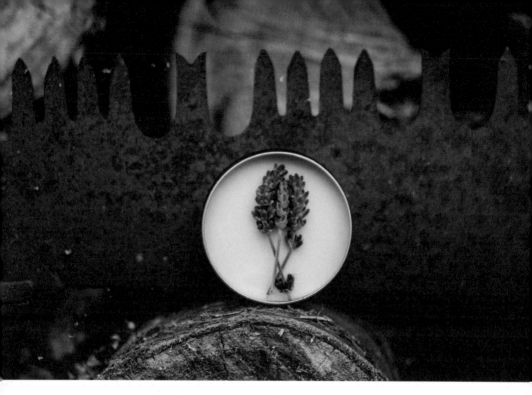

The Art of Self-Care

Lumberjack Beard Balm

This beard balm, crafted with the help of my husband, combines the ruggedness of a lumberjack with the soothing, calming, and refreshing aromatherapy properties of lavender, bergamot, and lime. He chose this fragrance combination for the memories it evokes from our wedding day, the oil and shea butter blend to leave his beard soft and manageable, and vitamin A to nourish his beard and the skin underneath. It's perfect for the wash-and-run type, as it takes just seconds to apply, and the essential ingredient, beeswax, provides the structural integrity needed for styling. This balm is the perfect companion for the bearded gentleman seeking to add a touch of nature to his daily routine.

Lavender-Infused Oil Ingredients

lavender, dried (amount will vary depending on size of storage container)

jojoba oil (amount will vary depending on size of storage container)

To Create the Oil

1. Fill a clean, dry glass jar three-quarters full with dried lavender buds. Pour in olive oil, completely covering the herbs. Use a clean wooden chopstick or skewer to move the herbs around to release any air bubbles.
2. If the lid to the jar is metal, place two small squares of parchment or wax paper between the mouth of the jar and the lid to prevent the metal from eroding. Alternatively, use a plastic screw top lid. Screw the lid tightly closed. Shake well.
3. Store in a cool dark place for four to six weeks, shaking daily.
4. Strain the plant material from the oil with a cheesecloth and fine screen strainer and store in an airtight glass jar for up to one year.

Beard Balm Ingredients

½ cup (115 g) beeswax pastilles

½ cup (115 g) shea butter

½ cup (120 ml) coconut oil

½ cup (120 ml) lavender-infused jojoba oil

10 drops vitamin E

5 drops lavender essential oil

15 drops bergamot essential oil

40 drops lime essential oil

Other essential and/or oil infusions that are appropriate for this recipe: cedar, frankincense, juniper, pine, sandalwood, sweet orange, tangerine, vanilla

To Create the Beard Balm

1. Combine the first three ingredients in a double boiler over low heat and stir occasionally with a disposable wooden chopstick or skewer until completely melted and combined.
2. Remove from heat and stir in the jojoba oil, vitamin A, and essential oils until combined.
3. Carefully pour the mixture into tins or clean, dry glass jars with airtight lids and leave undisturbed to cool to room temperature before moving or capping. This recipe yields seven 2-ounce tins.

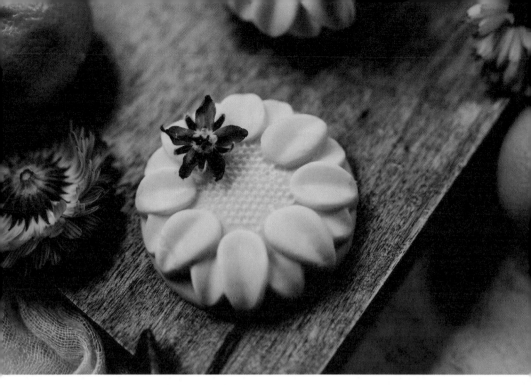

Calendula Borage Lotion Bars

Nourish your skin with these bars, packed with the soothing properties of calendula and the moisturizing benefits of borage. These compact bars are crafted to provide a convenient and mess-free way to hydrate and rejuvenate your skin, with a luxurious texture that melts upon contact.

Calendula Borage-Infused Oil Ingredients

calendula, dried (amount will vary depending on size of storage container)
borage, dried (amount will vary depending on size of storage container)

extra virgin olive oil or other carrier oil of choice (amount will vary depending on size of storage container)

To Create the Oil

1. Fill a clean, dry glass jar three-quarters full with the dried herbs. Pour in the oil, completely covering the herbs. Use a clean wooden chopstick or skewer to move the herbs around to release any air bubbles.

2. If the lid to the jar is metal, place two small squares of parchment or wax paper between the mouth of the jar and the lid to prevent the metal from eroding. Alternatively, use a plastic screw top lid. Screw the lid tightly closed. Shake well.
3. Store in a cool dark place for four to six weeks, shaking daily.
4. Strain the plant material from the oil with a cheesecloth and fine screen strainer and store in an airtight glass jar for up to one year.

Lotion Bar Ingredients

4 tablespoons (60 ml) coconut oil
½ cup (115 g) shea butter
¾ cup plus 1 tablespoon (187 g) beeswax

½ cup (120 ml) calendula borage-infused oil
1 teaspoon (5 ml) vitamin E oil
40 drops sweet orange essential oil
30 drops lavender essential oil

To Create the Lotion Bars

1. Combine the first four ingredients in a double boiler over low heat and stir occasionally until completely melted and combined.
2. Remove from heat, stir in the vitamin and essential oils and pour into silicone molds. Leave undisturbed for several hours until the bars are completely solidified.
3. Carefully remove them from the molds and wrap them in parchment paper secured with twine or a small piece of washi tape, or stack them in a glass jar with parchment paper between the bars.

Note: If the consistency of the bar is too soft for your liking, put them back in the double boiler to reheat to a liquid state and add another ¼ cup of beeswax. Remove from heat and add the essential oil combination again, as remelting can cause the oils to become less effective. Pour it back into the molds and leave undisturbed again until solidified.

To use, rub the bar directly onto your skin. The heat of your skin will melt the bar slightly, applying healing and replenishing properties.

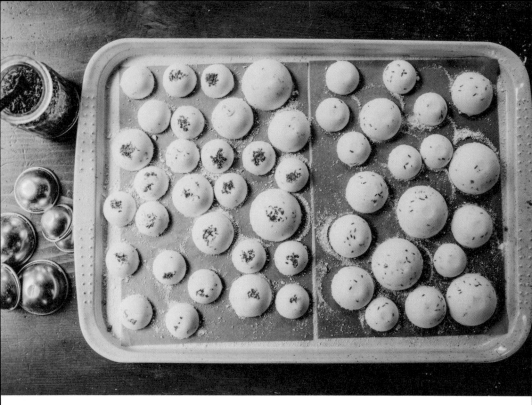

Rejuvenation Shower Steamers

As the days become shorter and the months begin to cool, I appreciate adding these homemade shower steamer varieties, Spearmint Lavender to decongest and soothe and Lemon Eucalyptus to revitalize my shower routine. The herbal combination of spearmint and lavender calms the senses and promotes relaxation while the combination of lemon and eucalyptus invigorates and awakens the senses. Indulge in these steamers to start your day on a rejuvenating note.

Ingredients

2 cups baking soda
1 cup citric acid
40 drops spearmint and 40
  drops lavender essential
  oils (or 40 drops lemon and
  40 drops eucalyptus)
witch hazel

lavender buds or lemon
  peel, dried (optional)

Specialty Supplies

metal bath bomb molds
misting bottle

To Create

1. In a bowl, mix the baking soda and citric acid until well combined. Add essential oils evenly around the bowl and mix until well combined.

2. Pour the witch hazel into a misting bottle and spritz it onto the mixture, beginning with 5 spritzes. Mix it quickly and then form it in your hand (like you're making a snowball) to test the consistency. If it falls apart, add another 3 spritzes and try again until you can form a ball that holds its shape. (The goal here is to use as little witch hazel as possible to obtain the necessary consistency. If it begins to fizz, it's too moist.)

3. Press the mixture into metal bath bomb molds, packing firmly to remove any air bubbles.

4. Carefully remove them from the molds and place them on a parchment-covered baking sheet for twenty-four hours.

5. When completely dry to the touch, stack in an airtight jar with small squares of parchment paper between each steamer and the next, or package individually in brown parchment paper and secure with twine.

257

Precautionary note: Use caution when using this product, as the oils can make certain bathtub surfaces slippery.

Note regarding dried plant material: this is an optional ingredient but is pretty and adds a lovely organic element to the steamers. There are two ways I incorporate dried elements into steamers. First, they can be added to the mixture in step 1. I recommend no more than two tablespoons (28 g) for each batch. Second, a pinch of your dried botanical can be added to the bottom of the metal mold before you spoon in your mixture. A pinch may seem like a small amount, but a little goes a long way with this recipe and too much dried botanical will negatively impact the structural integrity of the steamer. Less is more in this regard.

To use, place a steamer on your shower floor where the water will splash on it. As the steamer dissolves, its aromatic properties fill the air, transforming your shower into a spa-like oasis.

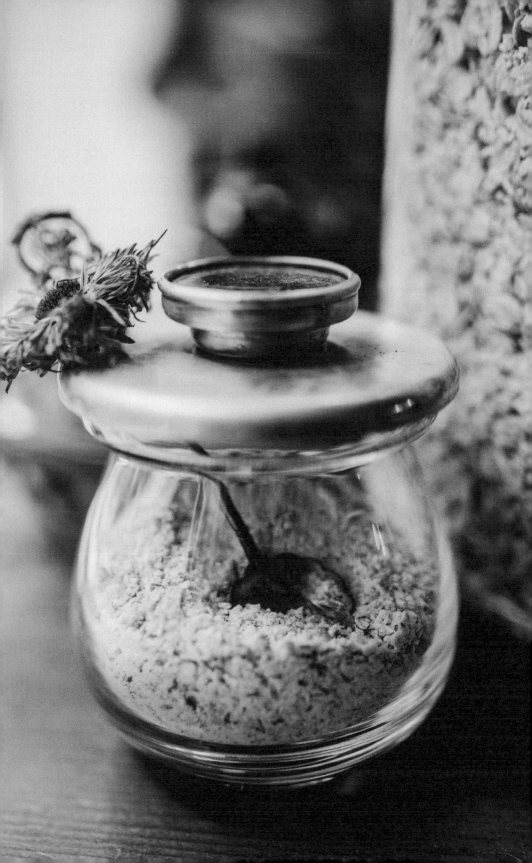

Calendula Chamomile Oatmeal Bath

I have struggled with eczema since I was a young girl and I've found that it flares up most during the winter months. This calendula oatmeal bath helps soothe dry, itchy winter skin and takes just minutes to make with ingredients you likely have around your home.

Ingredients

1 cup (227 g) calendula, dried
1 cup (227 g) chamomile, dried
1 cup (227 g) oatmeal
1 cup (227 g) baking soda
15 drops chamomile essential oil

15 drops mandarin
  orange essential oil

Specialty Supplies
4 muslin bags

To Create

1. Combine the first four ingredients using a food processor or blender until well blended.
2. Stir in essential oils.
3. Transfer to muslin bags and tie drawstring tightly closed or sprinkle directly into bath water.

To use, loop the drawstring of the muslin bag over your bath faucet or drop it into your bath, squeezing it every now and then to release the soothing properties into the water. The mixture can be stored in an airtight glass jar for up to six months.

> *Precautionary note:* Use caution when using this product, as essential oils can make certain bathtub surfaces slippery.

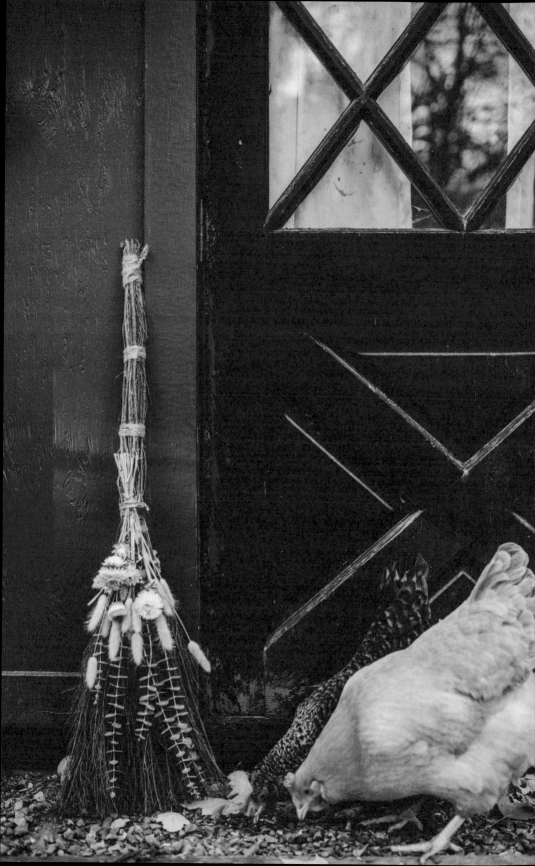

Garden-Made for the Home

Botanical Broomsticks

I ran across these cinnamon-scented broomsticks at my favorite market and instinctively popped a few in my cart. When I got home, I couldn't wait to try my hand at decorating them with dried botanicals I'd preserved from my garden. Dried eucalyptus, sage, cedar, strawflower, and a blend of bunny tails and other grasses are great options for an autumn-inspired broom. Add holly or mistletoe sprigs for a more festive broom to use and display during the winter months. Lean one on your living room hearth and use to keep the area around the fireplace tidy, one in your greenhouse to brush off your workbench, and one in the chicken coop to deodorize. At the end of the season, stow it away with your seasonal décor for next year or use it as kindling for your final fire of winter.

Ingredients

dried herbs and other botanicals of choice

twig broom(s), thirty-inch tall or miniature six-inch handheld broom(s)

To Create

1. Tie the dried herbs and botanicals onto the head of the broom with a bit of twine, beginning with the longest herbs, wrapping the twine around twice, and then continuing to stack each shorter layer of herbs on top so each previous layer is visible.
2. Double-knot it in the back and leave a few inches on the ends of the twine. Tie the ends together to create a loop for hanging.

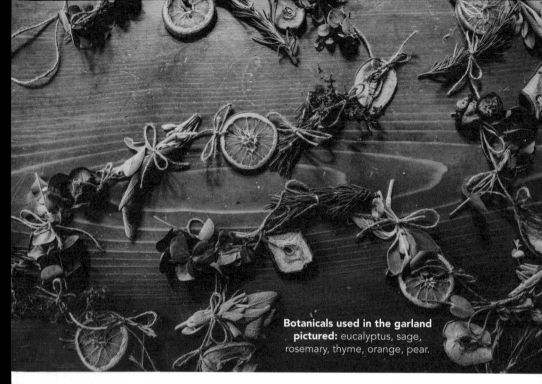

Botanicals used in the garland pictured: eucalyptus, sage, rosemary, thyme, orange, pear.

Herb and Orchard Garland

This craft beautifully intertwines my love for gardening, herbalism, and home décor. Herbs from our garden are tied to the garland alongside dried fruit from our small orchard. This garland can be used to decorate fireplace mantels, window frames, banisters, chicken coops, and barn doors, or strung to a fresh evergreen holiday wreath or Christmas tree. It will give several weeks of a lovely inviting fragrance, and the herb bundles can be easily untied from the twine to season your favorite savory dishes and drinks. While they hang, they naturally dry and can be preserved and used for the next twelve months. Preserved herbs tucked into pretty jars make beautiful and useful gifts too.

Ingredients

herbs of choice

fruit of choice, dried (pear, apple, and orange work well for this project)

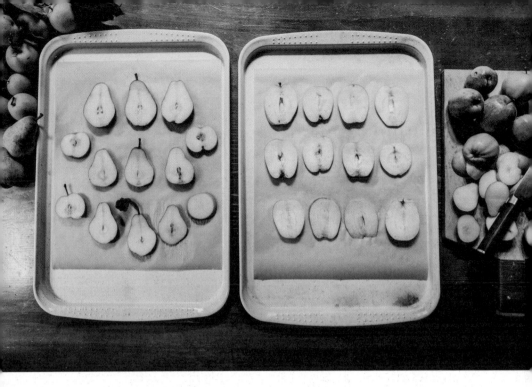

To Create

1. Slice fruit less than ¼-inch thick. The slices will be various diameters, which add character to the garland.

2. Line the fruit up on a parchment-lined cookie sheet and bake at 175 degrees F for two to three hours (or until the fruit is completely dried through). Alternatively, a dehydrator can be used.

3. While the fruit is drying, measure the space where you want to hang your garland and cut the twine to that length plus two feet, so the garland can hang down vertically about a foot on each end. Add a couple additional feet if you want the garland to drape along the top in a scallop formation. I have found that seven-foot-long garland strips are a good length for hanging in various spaces around my home.

4. Cut several nine-inch pieces of twine that will be used to attach your herbs and fruit to the primary twine. Cut more if you prefer your garland to be full and heavy with herbs. Cut less if you prefer a more simplistic look.

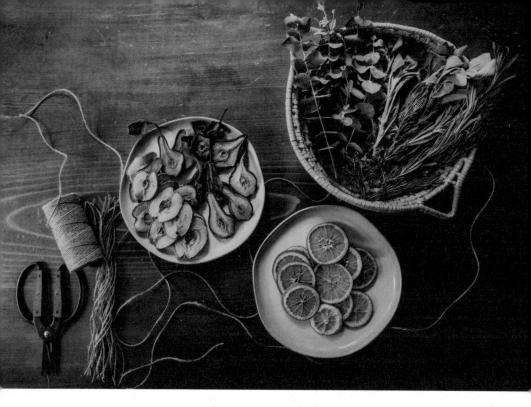

5. Cut the herbs into small bundles and tie them to your long piece of twine, spacing them out equally as shown. Secure them tightly, as herbs shrink as they dry.

6. Poke a hole near the top of each dried fruit slice and attach them using small pieces of twine, filling the spaces between the herbs. The herb bundles will slide back and forth with a gentle pull so you can reposition them as needed.

7. Add additional items to fit the season or your home's décor. Evergreen branch clippings, cinnamon sticks, fresh cranberries, jingle bells, or simple natural wooden beads are some seasonal ideas.

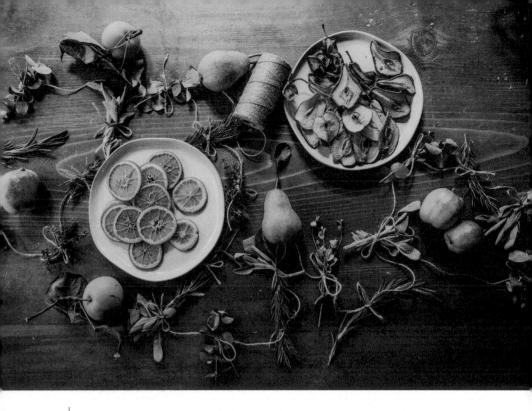

Autumn/Winter garland botanicals: cedar, eucalyptus, oregano, rosemary, sage, St. John's wort (leaves and berries), thyme

Spring/Summer garland botanicals: bee balm, calendula, chamomile, eucalyptus, feverfew, juniper (leaves and berries), lavender, lemon or lime wheels, mint, rose, sage, yarrow

265

Winter

"Winter is the time for comfort,
for good food and warmth,
for the touch of a friendly hand
and for a talk beside the fire;
it is the time for home."

—*Edith Sitwell* (1887–1964)

Heavy Blanket of Winter

A new year. A new chapter. A fresh start. Resolutions, if they suit you. Commitments to self-care or to learning something new. Perhaps you are a list-maker or a word-of-the-year chooser? Maybe you hang a new calendar or spend time decluttering your home. Whatever it is that shakes you awake when the calendar turns to January, I hope it includes an appreciation for herbs through crafting and creating. Incorporating herbs into your life is a conscious step toward a deeper connection with the earth and a slower, more intentional lifestyle. The culinary recipes that follow celebrate the winter season by using the dried herbs you've preserved this past garden season to add herbal notes to your favorite drinks and dishes. The self-care and home products encourage you to open your dried herb jars and uncap your oils, releasing the preserved energies from your summer garden. Several of these recipes also provide natural support to your home and family as you usher in the new year.

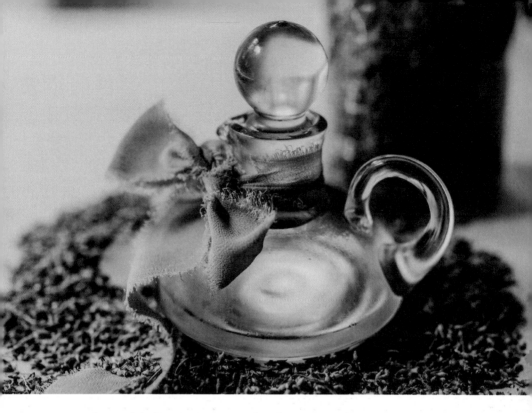

In the Kitchen

Herbal Simple Syrups

True to the name, herbal simple syrups consist of just three ingredients and take mere minutes to make. They are a staple ingredient in nearly every botanical craft cocktail I make, and a fantastic way to add depth and incorporate herbal hints and seasonal flavors into hot and cold mixed drinks. Once you understand the basic structure behind these elixirs, it will open the garden gates to endless variations of botanical flavors to elevate your craft cocktail creations.

Ingredients

1 cup (227 g) granulated sugar
1 cup (240 ml) filtered water

¾ cup (172 g) fresh herbs of
choice (or 1 cup [227 g] dried)

To Create

1. Combine the sugar and water in any one-to-one ratio and bring to a simmer over medium heat in a small saucepan, stirring often. (If you are adding fruit or spices to your syrup, add them now.)

2. Once your sugar is dissolved, stir in the herbs and simmer one more minute.
3. Turn heat off, cover, and let the syrup steep to room temperature.
4. Fine-strain into a clean glass jar, cover, and refrigerate.

Note: Simple syrup lasts approximately five days when kept sealed and refrigerated. To extend the life up to two weeks, stir in one tablespoon of vodka once it has cooled to room temperature but before refrigerating.

My Simple Syrup Potions

Beez Kneez—lavender, lemon balm

Earth Song[10]—rosemary, sage, and thyme

Floral Fusion[11]—borage, lavender, rose

Scarborough—parsley, sage, rosemary, thyme

Lavender—lavender

Lime Thyme—lime thyme (or common/German) plus peel from 1 lime

Mint—mint of choice

Rose—rose petals, packed

Secret Garden—rose, rosemary, thyme

Pearadise Sage—sage, sliced pear, teaspoon (5 ml) of vanilla extract, or ½ vanilla bean, split open

Yuletide—rosemary, juice and peel of 1 orange, 1 cinnamon stick, a small handful of cranberries, brown sugar

---

10 Add a single purple butterfly pea flower to naturally color your syrup a gorgeous green hue, to fit the earthy theme.

11 Add a single blue butterfly pea flower to naturally color your syrup a gorgeous blue hue, which will turn purple when mixed with most juices.

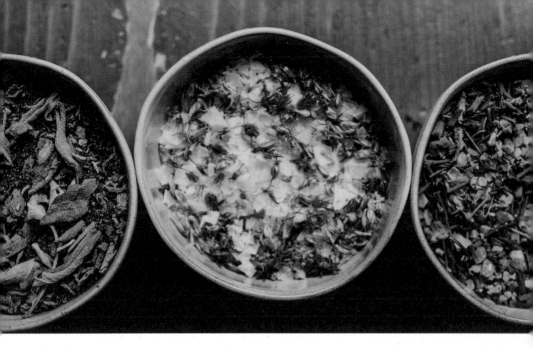

Herbal Finishing Salts

Herbal finishing salts combine the natural flavors of dried herbs with the versatile seasoning properties of salt, creating blends that, over time, meld together and infuse the salt crystals. The result is a visually appealing and aromatic seasoning that adds depth and complexity to a wide range of savory dishes. As a general rule, incorporate equal parts salt and herbs to create balanced blends that provide a burst of flavor. I use primarily coarse sea salt, though some combinations below call for smoked, pink Himalayan or Celtic Sea salts, each which have slightly different flavors or hues. Use the combinations below as a starting point and experiment with the ingredients to fit your own flavor preferences.

Ingredients

½ cup (115 g) salt

½ cup (115 g) dried herbs and other ingredients

To Create

1. Combine all ingredients in a bowl, using the one-to-one ratio of salt to herbs and other ingredients. If you are adding a flavored oil, two to three drops for every ½ cup (115 g) of salt is a good starting point. Stir to combine.

2. If you would like a finer consistency, blend the salt and herbs in a food processor, blender, or coffee grinder for a few seconds. Or omit this step and keep the salt at the original coarseness.

3. Funnel your salt into a clean, airtight glass container. Over time, the salts will absorb the flavor and aromatic profiles of the herbs.

To use, sprinkle a light amount of the finishing salts on dishes you wish to enhance. While finishing salts are typically added after dishes are prepared, they can also be used as a salt substitute in recipes and are wonderful additions to dressings and marinades. I particularly enjoy adding herbal finishing salts to my morning eggs, popcorn, and pretty much anything that is headed to the grill.

> *Note:* This recipe calls for dried herbs that will be more readily available to you during the winter months; however, if you are making this recipe during the spring or summer months and would prefer to use fresh herbs, simply spread the salt mixture on a parchment paper-lined baking sheet after step 2, and let it dry for one to three days, stirring occasionally, until fully dry.

271

My Favorite Herb Finishing Salt Combinations

Chive Florette—chive blossoms, sea salt

Rosemary+Lavender—rosemary leaves, lavender buds, sea salt

Calendula+Chive—calendula petals, chive leaves, sea salt

Florence—basil, black truffle oil, sea salt

Rose+Peppercorn—rose petals, coarse peppercorns, pink Himalayan salt

Savory Blend—oregano leaves, sage leaves, thyme leaves, rosemary leaves, sea salt

Lemon Sage—sage leaves, lemon balm leaves, dried lemon peel, sea salt

Tuscany—lavender buds, sage leaves, garlic flakes, sweet marjoram leaves, black pepper, Celtic sea salt

Smoke+Sage—sage leaves, smoked sea salt

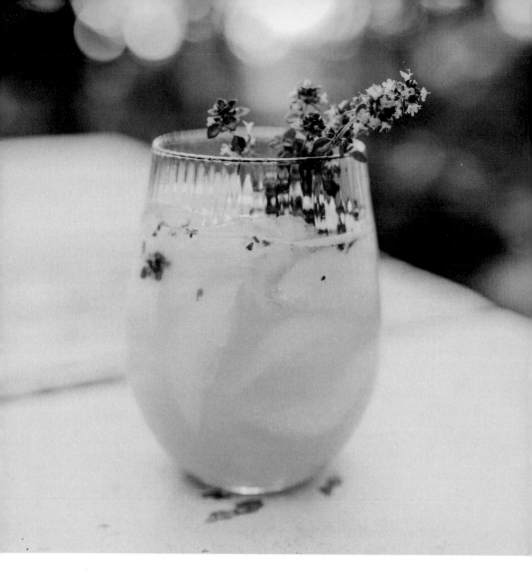

Seasonal Sips

Smoke + Thyme Serenade

The smoky allure of mezcal collides with the vibrant flavors of grapefruit and lime and earthy thyme notes in this exquisite libation. Then, the depth and complexity of the earthy thyme flavor makes this drink a sophisticated refreshment sure to be a crowd pleaser. If you have overwintered your thyme plants by bringing them inside during the winter months, you will be able to snip from them to add fresh sprigs to garnish this cocktail; however, a sprinkle of dried thyme also works well.

Ingredients

2 ounces (60 ml) mezcal

¾ ounce (22.5 ml) lime juice

1 ounce (30 ml) grapefruit juice

½ ounce (15 ml) lime
  thyme simple syrup

6 fresh common (German)
  thyme sprigs for muddling

champagne or Prosecco to
  top (a generous splash)

6 fresh lime thyme sprigs to garnish

To Create

1. Create the lime thyme simple syrup according to the recipe on page 269.
2. Combine the first five ingredients in a shaker with ice and shake vigorously for fifteen seconds until well-chilled.
3. Loosely strain over ice, so that the thyme stems are withheld but small pieces of the thyme leaves that were shaken off remain in the finished drink.
4. Top with a generous splash of champagne or Prosecco.
5. Garnish with a tiny bundle of fresh lime (or lemonade) thyme. (I bundle five sprigs together and tie them at the base with the sixth sprig.)

273

Note: Experiment with other simple syrup and herb combinations when concocting this cocktail. Other herbs that would complement the smokiness of the mezcal without being overpowered by it are sage, rosemary, and lemon balm.

Note: To make this cocktail a mocktail, omit the mezcal and champagne and add 4 ounces (120 ml) of your favorite flavored soda water or nonalcoholic tequila spirit substitute and a drop of liquid smoke.

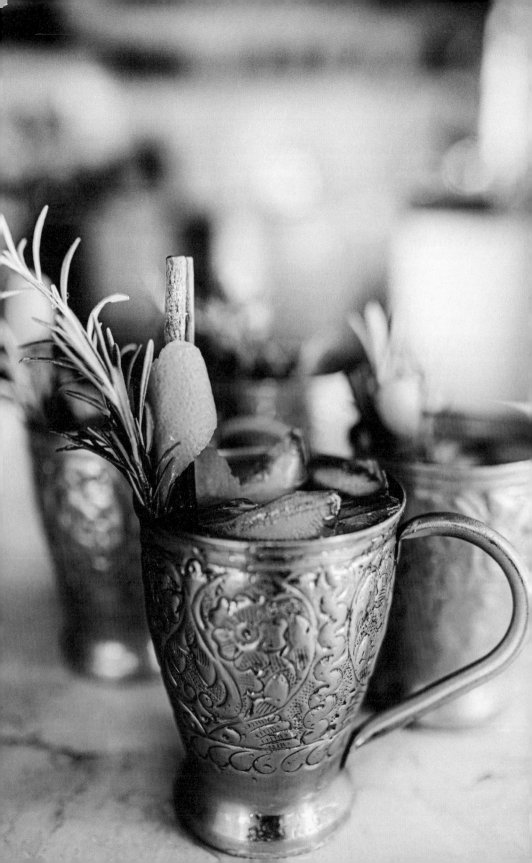

Holly Jolly Mule

I created this festive version of the Moscow Mule to serve at our annual Christmas party a few years ago, and it quickly became an annual tradition. It's easy to make, doesn't require shaking or muddling, and is guaranteed to break the ice and have everyone rockin' around the Christmas tree in no time.

Ingredients

2 ounces (60 ml) vodka, chilled

2 ounces (60 ml) cranberry juice, chilled

juice of ½ lime

½ ounce (15 ml) Yuletide simple syrup

ginger beer

To Create

1. Create the Yuletide simple syrup according to the recipe on page 269.
2. Fill a copper mug with ice.
3. Squeeze half a lime over the ice and compost the rind.
4. Pour the vodka, cranberry juice, syrup, and ginger beer over the ice.
5. Stir with a cinnamon stick and garnish with an orange peel twist and a sprig of rosemary that has been slapped on the table or clapped between your palms a time or two to release its aromatic properties.

Note: To make this cocktail a mocktail, simply omit the vodka.

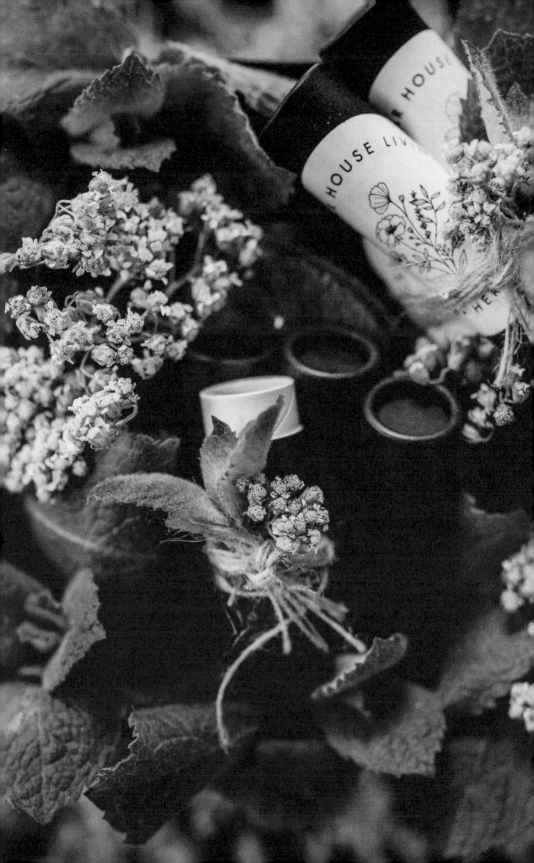

The Art of Self-Care

Healing Peppermint Lip Balm

Known for centuries as the "wound healer" for its skin healing abilities, yarrow is the key ingredient in this gentle but effective lip balm formula, crafted to soothe, heal, protect, and moisturize chapped lips. The peppermint adds a refreshing burst, awakening the senses and providing a cooling sensation.

Yarrow-Infused Oil Ingredients

yarrow, dried (amount will vary depending on size of storage container)

avocado oil (amount will vary depending on size of storage container)

To Create the Oil

1. Fill a clean, dry glass jar three-quarters full with the dried herbs. Pour the oil in, completely covering the yarrow. Use a clean wooden chopstick or skewer to move the herbs around to release any air bubbles.

2. If the lid to the jar is metal, place two small squares of parchment or wax paper between the mouth of the jar and the lid to prevent the metal from eroding. Alternatively, use a plastic screw top lid. Screw the lid tightly closed. Shake well.

3. Store in a cool dark place for four to six weeks, shaking daily.

4. Strain the plant material from the oil with a cheesecloth and fine screen strainer and store the oil in an airtight glass jar for up to one year.

Lip Balm Ingredients

1 cup (240 ml) yarrow-
  infused avocado oil
½ cup plus 2 tablespoons
  (143 g) beeswax pastilles

½ cup (115 g) shea butter
  or cocoa butter wafers
5 drops vitamin E oil
8 drops peppermint essential oil

Specialty Supplies

lip balm tubes or tins

Oil alternatives: sunflower, almond, olive, coconut

Essential oil alternatives: spearmint

To Make

1. Combine the first three ingredients in a double boiler over low heat and stir occasionally with a wooden disposable chopstick or skewer until completely melted and combined.
2. Remove from heat and stir in the vitamin and essential oils.
3. Using a narrow-mouthed funnel, carefully pour the mixture into tubes or tins and leave undisturbed to cool completely at room temperature before moving or capping.

Note: The amount yielded by this recipe can be easily adjusted. Just be sure the ratio is one part wax, one part butter, two parts oil, all by volume.

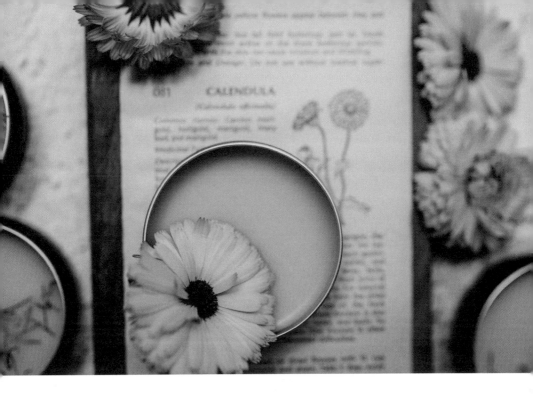

Calendula Salve

Calendula salve is a wonderful skin-care remedy to keep on hand, as it can help soothe eczema-prone dry skin, rashes, bug bites, minor cuts and scrapes, and minor burns. It is versatile and gentle enough for all ages to use, making it ideal for gifting as well.

Calendula-Infused Oil Ingredients

calendula, dried (amount will vary depending on size of storage container)

extra virgin olive oil (amount will vary depending on size of storage container)

sunflower or coconut oil, or blend of both (amount will vary depending on size of storage container)

To Create the Oil

1. Fill a clean, dry glass jar with dried calendula. Blend the oils together in a small bowl and pour over top of the dried flower heads, completely covering them. Use a clean wooden chopstick or skewer to move the herbs around to release any air bubbles.

2. If the lid to the jar is metal, place two small squares of parchment or wax paper between the mouth of the jar and the lid to prevent the metal from eroding. Alternatively, use a plastic screw top lid. Screw the lid tightly closed. Shake well.

3. Store in a cool dark place for four to six weeks, shaking daily.

4. Strain the plant material from the oil with a cheesecloth and fine screen strainer and store the oil in an airtight glass jar for up to one year.

Other herbs that would be beneficial in this oil infusion: chamomile, eucalyptus, juniper, lavender, rose, yarrow

Calendula Salve Ingredients

8 ounces (240 ml) calendula-infused oil

2 ounces (60 ml) beeswax

½ teaspoon (2.5 ml) pure Vitamin E oil

10 drops lavender essential oil

10 drops sweet orange oil

To Create the Salve

1. Combine the first two ingredients in a double boiler over low heat and stir occasionally with a wooden disposable chopstick or skewer until completely melted and combined.

2. Remove from heat and stir in the vitamin and essential oils.

3. Carefully pour the mixture into tins or glass jars and leave undisturbed to cool completely at room temperature before moving or capping.

Note: This recipe can be adjusted to fit your own personal preferences. The essential oils can be substituted, and if you prefer a firmer salve than this recipe makes, simply reheat it back to a liquid state, add a couple more pinches of wax pastilles, and pour back into the molds. Keep in mind that remelting the mixture causes the essential oils to become less effective, so add the essential oil combination again after taking the mixture off heat. If you prefer a creamier salve, use the same reheating process, but add a tablespoon (15 ml) more oil.

Note: This recipe makes five two-ounce storage tins or glass jars with lids. The amount yielded by this recipe can be adjusted to fit your needs. Just be sure the ratio is two parts wax to one part oil, by volume.

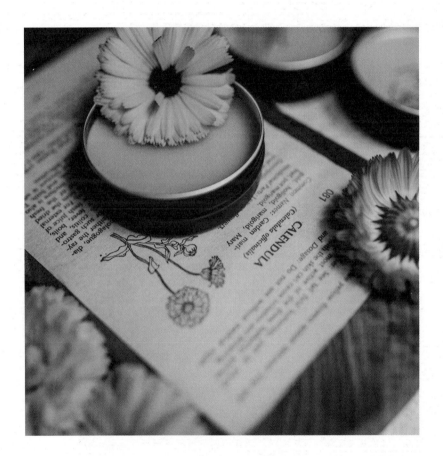

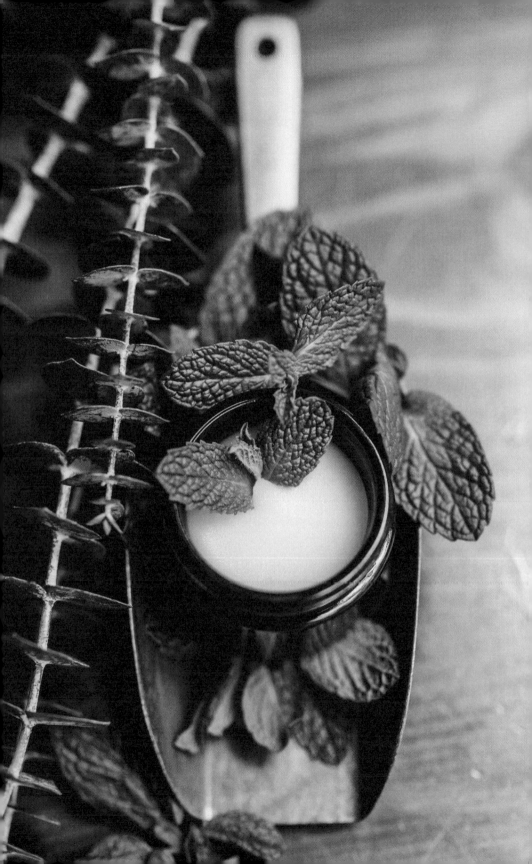

Breathe-Well Balm

During the cold and flu season, cough and congestion can be difficult to manage and can prevent you or someone you care about from getting a good night's sleep. This easy-to-make balm is great to have at the ready in your apothecary cabinet to bring quick relief without the use of chemicals. To use, apply to chest and bottom of feet as needed to relieve cough and congestion.

Ingredients

½ cup (120 ml) coconut oil (or almond oil)

2–3 tablespoons (28–42 g) beeswax pastilles

40 drops eucalyptus essential oil

40 drops peppermint essential oil

To Create

1. Combine the first two ingredients in a double boiler over low heat and stir occasionally with a wooden disposable chopstick or skewer until completely melted and combined.
2. Remove from heat and stir in the essential oils.
3. Carefully pour the mixture into amber jars (use a funnel) with plastic lids and leave undisturbed to cool completely at room temperature before moving or capping.

Precautionary Note: This recipe is for adults. Diluting the recipe by decreasing the essential oils to 20 drops eucalyptus essential oil and 20 drops peppermint essential oil and using minimally is commonly considered safe for children ages three and up; however, it is important to consult your health care professional before using any oils or herbs on your children. Never use on the face.

283

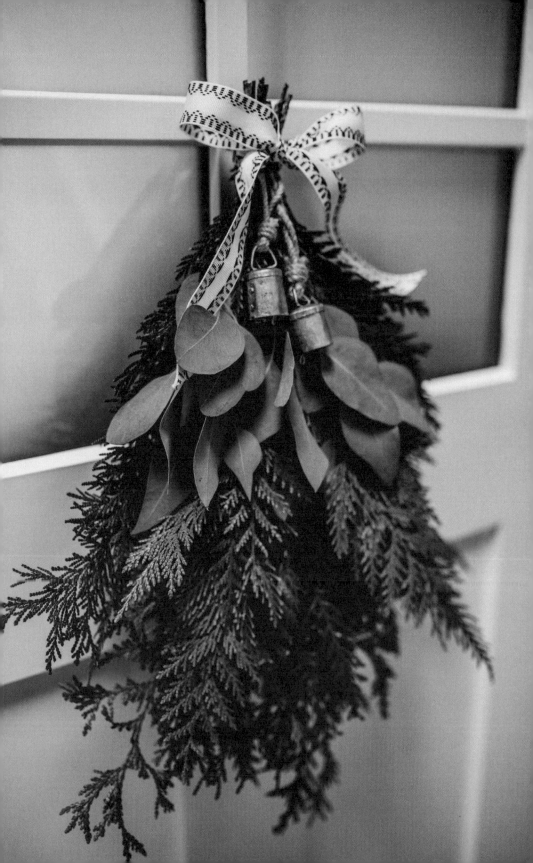

Garden-Made for the Home

Fresh and Foraged Cedar Swag

There's no lack of cedar boughs available on our property, so I put them to good use this year, making fresh cedar and eucalyptus swags as a fragrant alternative to a traditional wreath. These timeless, botanical bunches look beautiful adorning a door, hanging over the stove, or as a centerpiece on your holiday table. Representing strength and protection, cedar and eucalyptus are among my favorite botanicals to use for handmade wreaths, swags, and garlands.

Ingredients

8–10 fresh cedar boughs

fresh silver dollar eucalyptus sprigs, cut into small six-inch (15.24-centimeter) sections

Additional herbs that would be appropriate for this project: rosemary, peppermint

Additional herbs that could add a pop of color to this project: red rose, St. John's wort berries

Specialty Supplies

2 1.75-inch (4.45-centimeter) vintage gold bells on string

2- to 3-inch-thick (5- to 7.6-centimeter-thick) ribbon

To Create

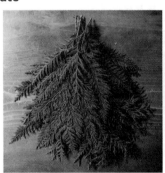 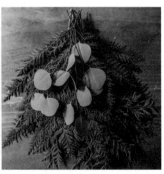

1. Gather eight to ten boughs of fresh cedar (Douglas fir, juniper, and white pine are other good options that may be readily available to you) and cut into sections approximately twelve inches long using garden shears.

2. Layer the boughs on top of each another, with the most widely sprayed ones in the back and the smallest ones in the front, holding the ends together at the top with one hand the entire time and shaping the swag into a fan shape.

3. While continuing to hold the ends of the cedar, add six-inch (15.24-centimeter) sprigs of eucalyptus, aligning the ends to the ends of the cedar. Two to four sprigs is usually a good amount.

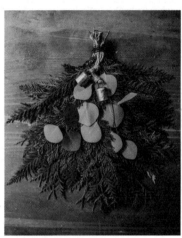 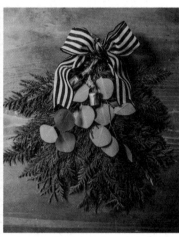

4. Loop the string of one bell over the botanical stem ends, weaving it through the ends and pulling downward to secure. Loop the string from a second bell over the stem ends twice so that it hangs slightly higher than the other.

5. Using green floral wire, tightly wrap the bell strings and the ends of the botanicals together. Tie a loop of floral wire in the back for easy hanging. Twist the ends of the wire together and tuck in securely.

6. Cut the ends of the plant stems to the same length for a clean, uniform look.

7. Finish with a thick ribbon bow to cover the floral wire and give your swag the perfect finishing touch.

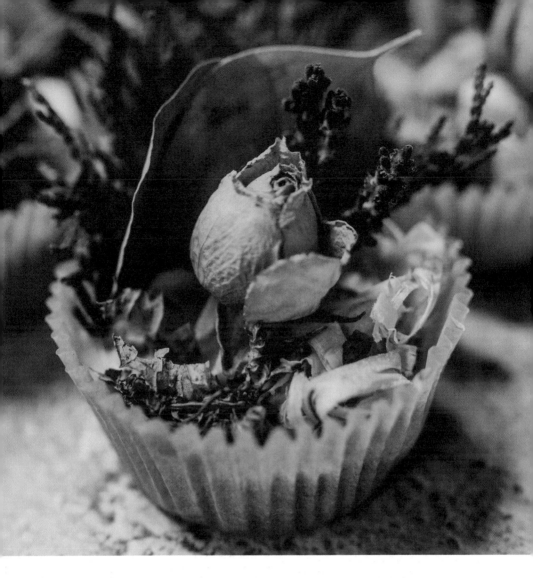

Botanical Fire Starters

Simple things made beautiful. These botanical fire starters give me the opportunity to rummage through my apothecary shelf and kitchen pantry to pull dried herbs that have expired or are discoloring. My youngest son, who loves counting and organizing, was in charge of placing the muffin liners in the tins and adding all the contents into each liner before I poured the wax. He was also charged with foraging wind-blown cedar branches and tiny pine cones from around the property. My favorite organic dried botanicals to gather for this project are eucalyptus, cedar, lavender, sage, mint, rose, and rosemary. My favorite spices to add are cinnamon sticks, star anise, whole cloves, and dried orange or lemon peel.

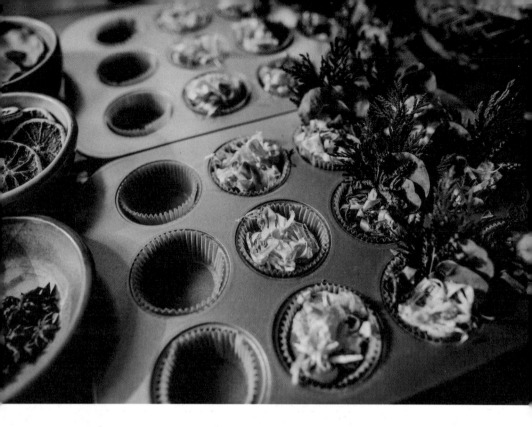

Ingredients

3 cups (682 g) organic
  beeswax pastilles
wood shavings (I use the pretty
  wood curls collected from
  my husband's woodworking
  bench, but any type of wood
  shavings, chips, or even dry
  foraged twigs will do)

dried herbs and spices
foraged wind-blown tree debris

Recommended dried herbs for this project: bee balm, calendula, catnip, chamomile, eucalyptus, mint, oregano, rose, rosemary, sage.

Specialty Supplies

muffin tin(s)

paper muffin liners

> *Note:* Many fire starter recipes online require resin and candlewicks; however, in my experience neither of those ingredients is necessary. Because I like to keep my recipes as simple and achievable as possible, I've omitted both of those from this tried-and-true recipe.

To Create

1. Prepare your muffin tin(s) with natural paper muffin liners.

2. Collect your fresh and dried plant ingredients and arrange them in the liners. (Reserve your favorite ingredients to add as "topping" later on in the project.)

3. Using a double boiler to melt the beeswax. Once completely translucent, carefully drizzle it over the plant materials in each of the muffin liners; approximately 3 tablespoons (45 ml) worth in each liner. Fill three liners at a time, alternating between this step and the following one. Doing so will ensure that the wax doesn't begin to dry before you have a chance to add your "toppings."

4. Before your wax dries, add your favorite, most attractive herbs to the top, setting them into the wax so they adhere. For my fire starters, I reserved the star anise, rose buds, and tiny pine cones for last. Allow the starters to fully cool.

This recipe creates a twelve-pack of fire starters.

> Beeswax can leave quite a mess on your pots and utensils. To clean them, melt the wax over low heat and then quickly wipe away the waxy residue with a paper towel. Lastly, wash with soap and hot water.

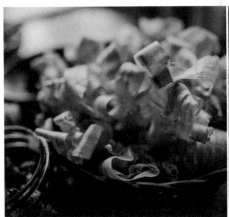
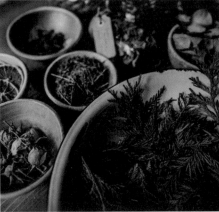

Acknowledgments

Many of the ideas for this book have grown based on my studies with the Herbal Academy, and the continuous inspiration from the herbal community, particularly my dear friend, Cat Seixas. It is also with a grateful heart that I acknowledge my editor, Lisa McGuinness, for her enthusiasm, commitment, and keen eye for detail as this book came to fruition, and Elina Diaz for her flawless design of the book. But none of this could have happened without my husband, Adam, and three children, Jack, Maddie, and Henry, who have given me endless support and patience while recipes and photography flatlays for this project were sprawled along our dining table more times than I could count, or when my attention was preoccupied with "just jotting down this one thought" for months on end. You graciously allowed me the time I needed to deepen my herbal knowledge and to develop this book to its full potential, even when it meant other tasks went to the wayside. You are my heart and my constant inspiration, and I am forever thankful for you.

About the Author

Jess and her husband, Adam, and three children live in a small town nestled in the mountains outside of Seattle, Washington. Their homestead, Cedar House Farm, is her sanctuary where she enjoys gardening, herbalism, farming, baking, writing, and photography. Jess is most at peace alongside her family and surrounded by botanicals.

Jess is an author and professional photographer. Her first book, *The Love Language of Flowers*, coauthored with Lisa McGuinness, is a botanical resource featuring three glossaries of flowers and their Victorian meanings, floriography, floral poetry and lore, and step-by-step instructions for creating impactful yet achievable arrangements infused with vintage meaning. It is available on Amazon and through most book retailers.

Jess has written pieces for several publications, including *Click Magazine, In Her Garden, Trailblazher Magazine, Willow & Sage, The Natural Home, GreenCraft*, and *Obaahima Magazine*. Her photography, recipes, and tutorials have been featured in various education resources offered by her friends at Herbal Academy, and her photography has been featured in National Geographic's *Your Shot USA, Your Shot UK,* and *The Daily Dozen*, among many other online photography publications. She was named one of the *Top 100 Photographers to Watch* by Click & Co. (2018) and is a Click Pro Elite Member and Click & Co. Lifetime Member. Her photography has been displayed in various exhibits and themed collections over the years.

Jess shares her botanical journey at instagram.com/cedarhouseliving and cedarhouseliving.com.

Works Consulted

Bennett, R. R. The gift of healing herbs; Plant medicines and home remedies for a vibrantly healthy life. Berkeley, CA: North Atlantic Books, 2014.

Bove, M. An encyclopedia of natural healing for children and infants (2nd ed.). Chicago, IL: Keats Publishing, 2001.

Castleman, M. The new healing herbs: the essential guide to more than 125 of nature's most potent herbal remedies (3rd ed.). Emmaus, PA: Rodale, Inc., 2009.

Cech, R. Making plant medicine (4th ed.). Herbal Reads LLC, 2016.

Chevallier, A. The encyclopedia of medicinal plants. DK Publishing, 1996.

Chevallier, A. Encyclopedia of herbal medicine: 550 herbs loose leaves and remedies for common ailments. DK Publishing, 2016.

Cornell University. Eucalyptus. http://bhort.bh.cornell.edu/histology/, 2013.

Daiki, J., Y. Kimura, M. Tamiguchi, M. Inoue, & K. Urakami. Effect of aromatherapy on patients with Alzheimer's disease [abstract]. Psychogeriatrics, 9, 173–179., 2009.

Edwards, G. F. Opening our wild hearts to the healing herbs. Ash Tree Publishing, 2000.

Ehrlich, S. D. Lemon balm. University of Maryland Medical Center, 2011.

Ellis, S. P. The botanical bible: Plants, flowers, art, recipes & other home remedies. New York, NY: Abrams, 2018.

Foster, S., & Duke, J. A. A field guide to medicinal plants and herbs of Eastern and Central North America. Houghton Mifflin Company, 2000.

Foster, S. Herbal Renaissance. Peregrine Smith Books, 1993.

Foster, S., & Johnson, R. L. National Geographic desk reference to nature's medicine. National Geographic Society, 2008.

Gardner, Z., & McGuffin, M. American Herbal Products Association's botanical safety handbook (2nd ed.). CRC Press, 2013.

Gladstar, R. Herbal remedies for vibrant health: 175 teas, tonics, oils, salves, tinctures and other natural remedies for the entire family. Storey Publishing, 2008.

Gladstar, R. Medicinal herbs: A beginner's guide. North Adams, MA: Storey Publishing, 2012.

Grieve, M. A modern herbal. New York, NY: Dover Publications, 1931.

Groves, M. N. Grow your own herbal remedies: How to create a customized herb garden to support your health and well-being. Storey Publishing, 2019.

Groves, M. N. Light in the darkness: Herbs to lift the spirits and support mood. 2019.

Hartung, T. Homegrown herbs: A complete guide to growing, using, and enjoying more than 100 herbs. North Adams, MA: Storey Publishing, 2015.

Herbal Academy. https://theherbalacademy.com, 2023.

Herbal Academy, Botanical mixed drinks recipe book: 82 cocktails & mocktails inspired by the seasons. Bedford, MA: Herbal Academy, 2023.

Herbal Academy, Botanical skin care recipe book: Featuring 194 favorite tried-and-tested herbal skin care recipes. Bedford, MA: Herbal Academy, 2019.

Hoffmann, D. Medical herbalism: The science and practice of herbal medicine. Healing Arts Press, 2003.

Johnson, R. L., Foster, S., Kiefer, D., & Low Dog, T. National Geographic guide to medicinal herbs: The world's most effective healing plants. National Geographic, 2012.

Kimmerer, R. W. Braiding sweetgrass: Indigenous wisdom, scientific knowledge, and the teachings of plants (2nd ed.). Minneapolis, MN: Milkweed Editions, 2020.

Kowalchik, C., Hylton, W. H. Radale's illustrated encyclopedia of herbs. Emmaus, PA: Rodale Press, Inc., 1987.

Mars, B. The desktop guide to herbal medicine: The ultimate multidisciplinary reference to the amazing realm of healing plants, in a quick-study, one-stop guide. Basic Health Publications, Inc., 2014.

McBride, K. The herbal kitchen. San Francisco, CA: Conari Press, 2010.

McIntyre, A. Flower power. New York, NY: Henry Holt and Company, 1996.

McVicar, J. Herbs for the home: A definitive sourcebook to growing and using herbs. New York, NY: Penguin Group, 1994.

Mojay, G. Aromatherapy for healing the spirit. Rochester, VT: Healing Arts Press, 1997.

Moradkhani, H., Sargsyan, E., Bibak, H., Naseri, B., Sadat-Hosseini, M., Fayazi-Barjin, A., & Meftahizade, H. Melissa officinalis L., a valuable medicine plant: a review. Journal of Medicinal Plants Research, 4(25), 2753–2759., 2010.

Mountain Rose Herbs https://mountainroseherbs.com, 2023.

Ody, P. The complete medicinal herbal. New York, NY: Skyhorse, 2017.

Pemberton, J. H. Roses: Their history, development, and cultivation. Bedford, MA: Applewood Books, 1920.

Pursell, J. J. The herbal apothecary: 100 medicinal herbs and how to use them. Portland, OR: Timber Press, 2015.

Stewart, A. The drunken botanist: The plants that create the world's great drinks. Chapel Hill, NC: Algonquin Books of Chapel Hill, 2013.

Stuart-Smith, S. The well-gardened mind: the restorative power of nature, New York, NY, Charles Scribner's Sons Publishing Company, 2020.

Tilth Alliance. Maritime Northwest garden guide: planning calendar for year-round organic gardening (2nd ed.). Seattle, WA: Tilth Alliance, 2014.

293

Herbal Utility Index

"To plant a garden
is to believe
in tomorrow."

—Audrey Hepburn

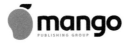

Mango Publishing, established in 2014, publishes an eclectic list of books by diverse authors—both new and established voices—on topics ranging from business, personal growth, women's empowerment, LGBTQ studies, health, and spirituality to history, popular culture, time management, decluttering, lifestyle, mental wellness, aging, and sustainable living. We were named 2019 *and* 2020's #1 fastest growing independent publisher by *Publishers Weekly*. Our success is driven by our main goal, which is to publish high-quality books that will entertain readers as well as make a positive difference in their lives.

Our readers are our most important resource; we value your input, suggestions, and ideas. We'd love to hear from you—after all, we are publishing books for you!

Please stay in touch with us and follow us at:

Facebook: Mango Publishing
Twitter: @MangoPublishing
Instagram: @MangoPublishing
LinkedIn: Mango Publishing
Pinterest: Mango Publishing
Newsletter: mangopublishinggroup.com/newsletter

Join us on Mango's journey to reinvent publishing, one book at a time.